Developments in Infant Observation

Infant observation was first introduced at the Tavistock Clinic by Esther Bick in 1948 and was devised by her as a method of assessing the development within the family of babies from birth to 2 years. Initially used only in the training of child psychotherapists at the Tavistock, the practice has now been adopted by child psychotherapists and other professionals all over the world and is the subject of many academic studies.

Studying a child within the home demands commitment from both observer and family, but the setting provides the intimacy through which the cognitive and emotional development of a particular child can be carefully and sensitively assessed. This pragmatic method differs fundamentally from the reading of texts on child development; observers are encouraged to see and 'feel' rather than simply to learn and attempt to apply theory. Infant observers are thus exposed to a new level of perception of human relationships that is both disturbing and exciting.

In 1993 the first ever International Conference on Infant Observation was held in London, and this book comprises eleven contributions selected and edited to provide an invaluable summary of the most recent theoretical developments and research initiatives in the field. Detailed material illustrates how the theories behind infant observation are put into practice, and helps to elucidate some of the more complex concepts for practitioners who may be unfamiliar with the Tavistock method.

Susan Reid is Consultant Child and Adolescent Psychotherapist and Senior Tutor in Child Psychotherapy at the Tavistock Clinic, London. She is currently engaged in research in autism and is co-director of a pilot research project on infant observation.

This book is dedicated to all the families who have so generously allowed us into their homes, and to the memory of Esther Bick, who originated this approach to infant observation.

Developments in Infant Observation

The Tavistock Model

Edited by Susan Reid

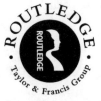

London and New York

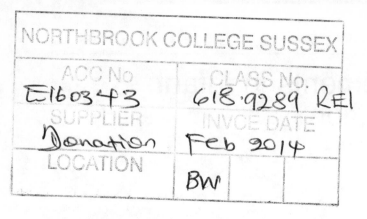
First published 1997
by Routledge
11 New Fetter Lane, London EC4P 4EE

Reprinted 1999

Simultaneously published in the USA and Canada
by Routledge
29 West 35th Street, New York, NY 10001

Routledge is an imprint of the Taylor and Francis Group

© the edited collection as a whole, Susan Reid; individual chapters, the
contributors

Typeset in Times by Intype London Ltd
Printed and bound in Great Britain by Creative Print and Design (Wales),
Ebbw Vale

British Library Cataloguing in Publication Data
A catalogue record for this book is available from the British Library

Library of Congress Cataloguing in Publication Data
Developments in infant observation: the Tavistock model / edited by
    Susan Reid.
        p.   cm.
    Includes bibliographical references and index.
    1. Infant psychiatry. 2. Observation (Psychology) I. Reid,
Susan, 1946– . II. Tavistock Clinic.
    [DNLM: 1. Child Development–congresses. WS 105 D4888 1996]
RJ502.5.D487 1996
618.92'89–dc20
DNLM/DLC
                                                              96–43621
                                                                   CIP

ISBN   0–415–14940–1 (hbk)
ISBN   0–415–14941–X (pbk)

Contents

Notes on contributors

Anne Alvarez is a Consultant Child Psychotherapist and co-convener of the Autism Workshop at the Tavistock Clinic. She helped to found the Observation Training course at the University of Turin and has taught on observation courses at Turin, Rome and Vienna. She has written widely on psychoanalytic topics and is the author of *Live Company: Psychoanalytic Psychotherapy with Autistic, Borderline, Deprived and Abused Children*. She is consultant to a research project in mother–infant psychotherapy for toddlers with Pervasive Developmental Disorders at the University of Pisa.

Olga Bazhenova was, at the time of writing her chapter with Alex Dubinsky, a Senior Researcher at the Centre for Mental Health at the Russian Academy for Medical Science and an Associate Professor of the Department of Medical and Neuropsychology in the Faculty of Psychology of the Moscow State University. She was a pioneer in infant observation in Russia, leading the first ever Infant Observation Seminar there. She is now a visiting scientist at the University of Maryland, USA.

Stephen Briggs is Senior Clinical Lecturer in Social Work in the Adolescent Department of the Tavistock Clinic. He is also Associate Senior Lecturer in the Department of Human Relations at the University of East London. He has a book in press entitled *Growth and Risk in Infancy*.

Gertraud Diem-Wille is a psychoanalyst working in private practice in Vienna, Austria. She is a lecturer at the University of Vienna. From 1992–3 she was a Visiting Scientist at the Tavistock Clinic.

Alex Dubinsky is a Child Psychotherapist, who trained at the Tavistock Clinic. He works in the National Health Service at the Child and Family Centre, Richmond Royal Hospital in Surrey. He teaches infant observation at the Tavistock Clinic and at the Centre Martha Harris in Larmor Plage, Brittany, France where he is Director of Studies. He was instrumental, with Dr Bazhenova, in instituting infant observation in the Faculty of Psychology at the State University of Moscow, Russia.

Lynda Ellis is training as a Child Psychotherapist at the Tavistock Clinic, and works as a member of a multidisciplinary child and family psychiatry team in Doncaster, England. She began her career as a social work practitioner specialising in therapeutic work with children and their families. In 1985 she became a Senior Lecturer at Sheffield Hallam University. She established the Family Studies Centre, a multidisciplinary forum aimed at improving ways of working together with children and families and was Director of the Centre for two years. She introduced child observation to social workers in training, and is co-author of a manual and video package introducing child observation training to the social work profession.

Piera Furgiuele is based in Turin, Italy. She is a Child Psychotherapist and teacher on the Child and Adolescent Psychoanalytical Psychotherapy Training Course organized by ASARNIA (Association for the Development of the Neuropsychiatric Relational Approach in Infancy and Adolescence), of which she is one of the founders and President. She is the author of several works on child psychosis, anorexia and borderline pathology during adolescence and work with parents.

Jeanne Magagna is a Consultant Child Psychotherapist heading the Psychotherapy Department for the Hospitals for Sick Children. She teaches on various trainings in Italy and England and works as a family and individual psychotherapist with people having severe communication and eating difficulties. She is also the joint coordinator of the Child Psychotherapy Training Programmes in Florence and Venice, Italy.

Suzanne Maiello is a Child Psychotherapist and adult analyst working in private practice in Rome, Italy. She is Organising Tutor for AIPPI – the child psychotherapy training in Italy. She also teaches infant observation in Berlin, Toulouse and Santa Fe. She has published widely on theoretical and methodological issues in psychoanalytic work with children and adults, with a special interest in research on pre-natal and early post-natal auditory experiences and their importance for psychic development.

Susan Reid is a Consultant Child Psychotherapist at the Tavistock Clinic where she is co-convener of the Autism Workshop and convener of the Group Psychotherapy Workshop. She is currently engaged in research in autism. She is a co-director of a pilot research project on infant observation.

Eric Rhode qualified as a Child Psychotherapist at the Tavistock Clinic, and worked in a hospital setting and in private practice. He is a Visiting Teacher at the Tavistock, where he teaches infant observation and seminars on the work of Wilfred Bion, and a training therapist at the London Centre for Psychotherapy and at the Association for Group and Individual Psychotherapy. Books on psychoanalytic topics include *On Birth and Madness, The Generations of Adam*, and *Psychotic Metaphysics.*

Maria Rhode qualified as a Child Psychotherapist at the Tavistock Clinic, and worked at the Hospital for Sick Children at Great Ormond Street and in private practice. She holds an academic post as Consultant Child Psychotherapist at the Tavistock, where she teaches on the clinical training for child psychotherapists. She is a training therapist at the London Centre for Psychotherapy and the Centre for Psycho-Analytic Psychotherapy, and has taught Infant Observation at the Tavistock and at the Lincoln Centre. Her other main interests are language delay, autism and psychosis in children.

Pamela Berse Sorensen is Assistant Professor of Psychiatric Medicine in the Department of Psychiatric Medicine at the University of Virginia Medical School where she is Director of the Under Fives Study Center. She teaches infant observation and child psychotherapy. She is also on the Faculty of the Washington School of Psychiatry.

Isca Wittenberg has introduced Infant Observation to trainings in a number of countries. For many years she was a Consultant Child and Adolescent Psychotherapist in the Adolescent Department at the Tavistock Clinic, and was Vice-Chair of the Clinic for ten years. She continues to teach at the Tavistock and in many countries around the world. She has published widely, including two books introducing other professionals to psychoanalytic thinking.

Preface

In 1948 Esther Bick introduced infant observation to the training of child psychotherapists at the Tavistock Clinic.

In 1992, during a training meeting with my child psychotherapy colleagues, our discussion turned to infant observation: it is a passion shared by us all. We had each been inspired, first by our own experiences of observing and then teaching infant observation to others, by the seemingly limitless source of ideas this provided. Whilst we relished any opportunity for discussion, it suddenly struck me that we had never really given ourselves the opportunity to explore and review the developments that had taken place in infant observation, the theoretical developments that had arisen from it, and the changes to clinical practice that it had informed. In fact we realised that, at the Tavistock where this fascinating approach to the study of the early development of the human species had begun, we had never held a conference on the subject. In September 1993 the first Tavistock Conference on Infant Observation duly took place. Limited space informed our decision to invite those people currently involved in the teaching of infant observation. We were over-subscribed and had members attending from twenty-one countries around the world.

The conference was an enormous success: papers were written specially for the occasion and generated stimulating discussions and a request for the conference papers to be brought together as a book. There was a quality of 'missionary zeal' amongst the membership, who wanted an opportunity to read and re-read the papers themselves at leisure. But also they wanted to have the ideas that had inspired us all, available in a form which could be shared with their own students around the world, and with their many colleagues who had been unable to attend.

The work of reshaping the papers to create a book accessible to all those people who want to know more about psychoanalytic infant observation, has been a slow and at times painful business. The gestation period for this book has more in common with that of the elephant than the human infant!

Some of the contributions to the conference have been impossible to include within this volume. A very moving and thought-provoking video presentation by Romana Negri, which opened our conference, cannot, for obvious reasons be included. However, the interested reader can now turn to Negri's book *The Newborn in the intensive care Unit: A Neuropsycho-analytic Prevention Model*, which was published in 1994. Similarly, contributions from different centres around the world, relating new developments in the practice and application of infant observation, could not be included in this volume for reasons of space. We hope they will find a well-deserved forum at a future date, if our aspirations to produce a journal of infant observation are realised. It is a great loss that the work of Kamala DiTella in Argentina cannot be represented in this volume due to her untimely death.

This compelling approach to the study of the early development of the human species has spread beyond anything that Mrs Bick could have imagined. Psychoanalytic infant observation has spread from its small beginnings as part of the child psychotherapy training at the Tavistock to many other psychoanalytic and psychotherapy trainings, to the trainings of other colleagues in the helping professions around the world. The last decade has seen a spurt of interest in the academic study of infant development and in the field of infant psychiatry. The burgeoning interest in infantile development has opened up the possibility of an exchange of ideas between clinicians, researchers and academics. In 1994, for example, a conference organised by sociologist, Professor Michael Rustin of the University of East London, was held at the Tavistock. The differences between the methodology described in this book and that of the attachment theorists, Mary Maine and Eric Hesse, were highlighted, and found to be mutually enriching.

Psychoanalytic concepts explored in this book are often complex, but the reader new to these ideas should be helped by the fact that the concepts used are often examined from different perspectives in several chapters. Although many of the concepts used are difficult, the infant observations not only stand as narratives in their own right, allowing us into a particular infant's world at a particular point in time, but also illuminate and elucidate some of the more complex ideas which the various authors are trying to develop.

The book is divided into three parts: to some degree these divisions are artificial since in many ways each chapter overlaps with others, not only in the same section but in other sections too. Nonetheless it is hoped that organising the book in this way will be of assistance to the reader. The chapters in Part I are primarily concerned with the actual practice of infant observation and therefore will form a useful basis for those unfamiliar with the method. Part II brings together all those chapters which explore new conceptual developments arising out of particular experiences in infant observation. Part III explores new developments in applying infant observation for the purposes of research. Each of the three sections is preceded by an introduction.

In the interests of confidentiality, names of the babies and their families have been changed throughout the book and identifying features removed. We have frequently used the term 'mother' in general discussion but it should be understood that this refers to whoever is the caregiver.

We hope that this book will be of interest, not only to those working psychoanalytically and to a wide variety of professionals in the helping professions, but also to colleagues who are engaged in academic and research studies in early development.

Reference

Negri, R. (1994) *The Newborn in the Intensive Care Unit: A Neuropsychoanalytic Prevention Model*, London: Karnac Books and Strath Tay, Perthshire: Clunie Press.

Acknowledgements

I have been supported throughout in the preparation of this book by Jane Rayner: her secretarial assistance, helpful comments as a 'lay reader' and encouragement have been invaluable.

Maria and Eric Rhode gave freely of their time in the early stages when difficult decisions had to be made about what could and could not be included, and I am particularly grateful to them. The work involved in bringing together the contributions of so many writers from different countries has been slow; at different stages many colleagues have offered practical support, advice and encouragement. I hope I will be forgiven if I have left anyone out. I would like to thank: Anne Alvarez, Pamela Gair, Trudy Klauber, Lisa Miller, Albert Reid, Margaret Rustin, Michael Rustin and Biddy Youell; and also Gill Ingall, Angela Haselton, Sheila Miller, Graham Shulman, Margot Waddell and Gianna Williams.

Finally, I would like to thank my family for their tolerance and support throughout.

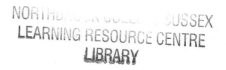

Chapter 1

Introduction

Psychoanalytic infant observation

Susan Reid

WHAT IS INFANT OBSERVATION?

This chapter is intended primarily for the reader who is not familiar with the practice of infant observation. A fuller discussion of the functions and theory of infant observation is to be found in *Closely Observed Infants* (Miller *et al.* 1989).

The psychoanalyst, Esther Bick, pioneered the practice of psychoanalytic infant observation in 1948. It became part of the training programme for those students studying to become psychoanalytic child psychotherapists (Bick 1964). Later, in the 1970's infant observation became part of a course of wider observational studies for many other professionals.

Each observation takes place in the baby's home; ideally the observer meets the parents before the baby is born, and then visits the family for an hour each week until the second birthday. As far as is possible, these hourly visits are at the same time of day each week. A parallel is made with psychoanalytic clinical work itself in that the observer is instructed not to take notes during the observation, but instead to record, in as much detail as can be recalled, all the events that took place during that hour. The emphasis in this method of observation is on what is seen and *felt* during the observation, and premature attempts to explain and make formulations are actively discouraged.

What is the impact then, of this open-minded, naturalistic observation? The student is encouraged and supported to *see what is there to be seen* and not to look for what they think should be there. Initially this may be an alarming experience since it strips the observer of the usual competences which protect each of us from being taken unawares; the observer has no idea what he or she will see and therefore is exposed to a whole new level of perception of human relationships. This is both disturbing and exciting.

Mrs Bick realised the training potential of this naturalistic method of infant observation. It has steadily spread so that most psychodynamic psychotherapy trainings in Great Britain include it as a central requirement. This very distinctive approach to studying the development of babies within the family has also rapidly spread to the training of others in the helping professions, such as social workers, clinical psychologists and doctors, not only in this country but around the world. The last twenty years have seen an enormous increase in the academic study of infant development and the work of researchers such as Brazelton (Brazelton *et al.* 1974), Stern (1985), Trevarthen (1976) and Main and Hesse (1992) can be seen to complement the findings of this method.

BECOMING AN OBSERVER

The start of an observation is difficult and disquieting for every observer. Each individual will have varying degrees and types of knowledge of how infants develop. Some will have a thorough grounding in theories of child development, some will already be parents themselves and thus will have had intimate contact with infants. Others will be experienced child care professionals. Each observer will of course, long ago, have been an infant, and although for most people conscious memories of the first two years of life are lost, these memories lie in waiting in the unconscious of each of us, ready to be evoked by intimate contact with the infantile experiences of another human being. It is well documented that parents find themselves deeply stirred by the experience of contact with their own infants. In most cases this can deepen their empathy with both the helplessness and the capacities of their own child – providing, that is, that they are not too emotionally overwhelmed by the experience and also have sufficient support in their own adult lives.

However experienced the new observer, beginning an observation is a great equaliser. It strips away much of what we thought we knew and exposes the ignorance and prejudices in each of us. To observe well, the observer has to relinquish their current professional identity. We discover how easy it is for activity in professional situations to mask anxiety and uncertainty, and even interfere with the best interest of our clients. We may also discover the liberation in thinking which follows upon the close attention to detail. It is likely to have a lasting influence on our subsequent professional lives when we discover how much an infant (and any other family member) responds positively to the experience of having our close attention upon them. We discover the real meaning of containment (Bion 1962), one of the most useful theoretical concepts ever developed to aid us in our understanding of what it is human beings need throughout life, in order to be able to function effectively. By adulthood, much of this capacity has been internalised – if we were fortunate in our caregivers in infancy. However, we continue to need containment by others at times of stress. We are always aware when someone is *really* attending to us, not merely going through the motions.

Containing another is a generous act, natural to the mother of the infant, unless she is emotionally overwhelmed herself. It means suspending temporarily our own needs and wishes in favour of those of another. It means putting our own mind at the disposal of another and, therefore, what we will be required to do for them may disturb our own equilibrium. Experiencing containment is to feel loved and cared for and may result in a responsive feeling of gratitude which initiates a loving or caring act in return. Sometimes gratitude is not felt because it is overwhelmed by envy; an envy of the capacity to do what we are unable to do ourselves. Where gratitude follows upon containment, then a benign cycle is set in place, supportive of healthy emotional development. Where containment is absent, or worse, the mother burdens the infant with her own unmet infantile emotional needs, then a pathological defensive system may be set up which arrests, or may pervert, healthy development.

The containment offered by the experience of being attended to closely is something we all know about; perhaps when a friend is able to listen and feel some distress of ours, and is able to bear knowing that they cannot change the external situation for us. What is changed, however, we know from experience, is our internal situation – we *feel* better. The external situation may well remain exactly the same but we *feel* differently about it. We are no longer alone and abandoned to distress, but have someone to share it with us. This experience is internalised and reinforces our sense of goodness in others and in ourselves. When the internal world is replenished in this way we, feeling sustained and nourished, may also find new resources to deal with a miserable situation. It may even shift our perspective, allowing us to discover, for ourselves, a new approach to the problem.

This is what underpins the psychoanalytic approach to therapy. Not the giving of advice, but the taking in, by the therapist, of everything that the patient needs to project at one moment in time. The act of thinking about, and feeling for, the patient may modify that projection, returning it in what Bion (1965) called a 'transformed condition'.

Professionals exposed to the psychoanalytic approach to infant observation can incorporate this understanding into their own professional practice. We learn the true value of attention and considered reflection, and to limit action mostly to moments of crisis where to be inactive would be to expose our clients to risk. It enfranchises the person with whom we are working, supporting that individual in discovering what is best for them.

Exposure to psychoanalytic infant observation also helps in selection and self-selection for psychoanalytic training, helping individuals to see whether the pain of seeing clearly is sufficiently balanced by the pleasure of new insights into human relationships. To observe in this way is like having scales removed from one's eyes – exciting and terrifying at the same time. It allows the possibility of generating new ideas and hypotheses, rather than looking for evidence to substantiate existing theories. It is an enormous shock for any observer to discover how little we really see, in ordinary situations, of what is going on. We see the surface of things, but not the deeper level of human interactions and communications. This is essential, of course, in the conduct of our daily lives. It is emotionally and intellectually demanding and exhausting to observe in the way I am describing. Indeed one might really say we were never intended to *see* in this way. Everyday relationships are essential to our survival – they probably cannot bear too close scrutiny – but for any professional working in the caring professions, the capacity for close and detailed observations (called upon in our different professional settings) makes us more effective in the service of our clients, pupils and patients.

THE ROLE OF THE INFANT OBSERVATION SEMINAR

Each observer is supported in this difficult endeavour by the seminar leader and other seminar members. Within an infant observation seminar group the teacher and seminar members are in a position to allow their attention to be free-floating and overarching, to travel back and forth in time. The observer, on the other hand, has been assiduously squirrelling away each nut of information and placing it in a time sequence in order subsequently to record a series of events observed. In this state of mind 'poetic intuitions' (see Eric Rhode, Chapter 5) can seem a mere distraction from the primary task. The seminar leader seeks to create a setting which allows space for appreciation of the actual observation, now firmly fixed on paper, and to support the free associations, ruminations and speculations of the observer and seminar members, to see what other dimensions remain to be discovered. This 'state of mind' of the seminar group is here analogous to the state of mind of the mother in 'reverie' (Bion 1962); making the distinction between a mindful mother and a mother who is only able to look after the baby's physical needs. The role of the seminar leader is here again analogous to the 'good mother' whose task, as I see it, is to provide those conditions which are necessary to allow the baby gradually to discover the world (with due regard to safety), and their place in it, and not just to teach the infant what she knows. This is what Bion calls 'learning from experience': not to fill the baby's mind up with the contents of her own, but rather to allow the infant to develop an original personality. Of course we all know that this is extremely difficult to do. Anxiety often pushes us to 'inform the seminar' (see Isca Wittenberg, Chapter 2), just as the mother can feel driven to inform or over-teach her infant, for fear that her child will not learn. Both mother and seminar leader fear that they will be revealed to be lacking. The state of mind necessary to allow the infant and seminar students to learn through the experience of personal discovery is optimistic, generous and hopeful.

There is pleasure to be found in the discovery that someone else will see events unfolding from a brand new perspective. This can engender real creativity; each individual builds up, in interaction with the outside world, their own internal world, unique to that individual. The discovery of another perspective has the potential, providing we are not over-whelmed by envy, to spark a fresh creation for each and everyone. It is the task of the seminar leader, just as it is the task of a mother, to create an environment in which it is possible for discovery to take place and for this to be a source of pleasure to all those concerned. Where mother or seminar leader becomes overwhelmed by anxiety there is a danger that growth may be crushed before it can flower. An example from an infant observation may illustrate this:

Mary enjoys a loving relationship with both parents. By the time she is almost 2 years old she is a confident, competent and creative little girl. Daddy has just arrived home and Mary wants him to play 'horsey'. Dad is obviously not keen but offers to play later. Mum suggests that she and Mary sit together on the floor to play with Mary's new plastic stacking cubes. The observer writes:

> Mum gently shows Mary the new cubes, telling her 'The red brick is the biggest, then the blue goes on next'. After a while Mum goes out into the kitchen to make Mary's supper, telling her what she is doing. Mary carries on building a tower; as she picks up each cube she says to it 'Is this one big?' or 'Is this one small?' She shows each cube to me (the observer) before putting it in its place. From time to time she experiments, putting a small cube inside a bigger one and leaving it there. When the tower is finished, she knocks it down with a flourish and says It fell down!' She is very amused by this. She then starts to build the tower again in just the same way, turning to look at me, very spontaneously and openly. At this point Mum comes back to see how Mary is getting on and points out the mistakes Mary has made in putting some small bricks inside big ones in building her tower. This time Mary smashes her tower with a sweep of her arm. She looks angry and confused. Mum looks slightly shocked and tells her off.

Mother unwittingly has crushed the baby's creativity, an incipient poetic construction, which she has developed upon what mother has shown her to be the 'properties of towers' and what, in the past, she has discovered with mother's support to be the 'properties of bricks'. On this occasion pleasure, delight, concentration and imagination are destroyed by a care-less comment from mother. Such careless comments, of course, are part of everyday life for any infant. No mother can be mindful of the baby's needs and creative capacities all the time.

For each infant, and for each seminar group, the innate nature of the infant, or group, will determine how soon they 'risk' creativity again. Here we can see, illustrated by Mary's response, the pleasure but risk involved in creativity, versus the pull to conformity. Will she in future only build a tower in the 'proper' way? Every new thought, idea or association produced by the seminar also has an element of risk attached to it. Each contribution is open to examination by the other seminar members, and each seminar member therefore needs to feel safe that their contribution will be dealt with respectfully.

WHY DO INFANT OBSERVATION?

Infant observation re-exposes each observer to the emotional roller-coaster that constitutes the experience of infancy for each of us when discovering the world and our place in it. It is a pragmatic method of studying child development and differs fundamentally from reading texts on theories of child development.

Observers can learn first, from the experiences of their own observations and second, from the observations of their fellow seminar members, about the impact of sexual identity, family position, social class, race, culture and different child-rearing practices, on infant development. It sensitises the group to the impact of the emotional atmosphere within which a baby lives and grows, no matter which of these factors prevail.

When observing an infant in the family we discover the intimate details of the pleasures and pains of physical, cognitive and emotional growth for a particular child. These experiences can then be compared with the experiences of other infants observed within the same seminar group, and in turn inform a reading of the various theories of child development. It makes the reading of theories more dynamic, more interactive. Each observation is a small research study in its own right: stirring and challenging the observer intellectually and emotionally. Any subsequent readings will therefore be in a more critical, reflective state of mind. Experiences from infant observation may therefore support us in challenging aspects of received wisdom – to change or add to a body of knowledge. Such critical faculties are essential for us all, whatever our professional background, if we are to develop our understanding of human nature. They are essential for psychoanalytic practitioners if we are to extend the range of our work and increase our effectiveness with our patients. Without them we would not have moved on from Freud's discoveries. Insights gained from infant observation have informed changes in technique, making it possible to work more effectively with patients who are hard to reach or who would previously have been considered unsuitable for psychoanalytical psychotherapy.

Sometimes not being able to *see* what is really happening is powerfully destructive of the emotional development and mental health of countless individuals. The Robertsons' observational films, made in the 1950s, have been influential in underlining the 'blindness' of society as a whole to the suffering and damage which lengthy, traumatic hospitalisations and separations could do.

The Robertsons' films reveal something so unbearably painful that there is a collusion not to see what is really there to be seen, *unless* the pain of seeing clearly can be channelled usefully. It becomes clear, then, that to observe in this way is to bear witness.

What one sees, observing human relationships closely, is often extraordinarily moving and beautiful but can be deeply upsetting and disturbing to one's own equilibrium. It can be compared to looking at human relationships through a microscope, focusing on the tiny details involved in any human exchange. Feeding an infant, for example, is revealed to be an extraordinarily involved exchange, whether the young infant is fed by breast or bottle. Infant and usually mother but sometimes father or another carer are involved in a multi-sensory exchange. We can observe that feeding involves the baby's mouth and mother's nipple (or the nipple of the bottle); baby's body and mother's body (or its absence where a baby is propped up in a pram or against pillows with a bottle); mother's arm and baby's hands; baby's eyes and mother's eyes; the smell of each for the other; the attention, or lack of it, of each for the other; mindfulness and absent-mindedness (Chapter 6); the mother's voice and the baby's vocal responses (Chapter 10); the prevailing atmosphere within which the feed takes place; the room or setting for the feed – is it calm and peaceful, or noisy and intrusive? It soon becomes clear that there is an infinite variety of ways in which a mother and baby can experience a feed, and that this experience goes way beyond the provision of milk by the mother, and the swallowing and digestion of it by the infant. The question to be asked then about the nature of a feeding experience becomes a much more complex and larger one; extending beyond whether a baby is bottle- or breast-fed and whether or not the baby is putting on weight. (It is perhaps more accurate to say that when the experience does not go beyond the mere provision of food then something is profoundly wrong. So wrong that, in the absence of provision of these other elements to the feeding situation, some babies give up and die; see Spitz 1946).

APPLICATIONS OF THE METHOD OF CLOSE OBSERVATION TO OTHER PROFESSIONS

Understanding the complex nature of the experience of the feed for mother and baby is crucially important for those who monitor the development of infants. The capacity for close observation can inform thinking about the reasons for particular difficulties and thereby guide decisions towards a helpful intervention.

Close and detailed observations using this naturalistic method allow the professional access to the internal and external world. They underline the individuality and uniqueness of each human being, and in doing so offer some protection from rigid, prescriptive thinking and adherence to particular ideologies, or unhelpful pressures from colleagues.

For the clinician, observations of infants feeding provide a unique source of information about the range of feeding experiences in early infancy. They allow for comparisons between infants and can therefore reveal those situations where we might expect an infant, in puberty or adolescence, to develop eating difficulties.

It will be apparent that, after fifty years of the exponential expansion of infant observation, the number of infant observations undertaken using this method probably now runs into the thousands. This is a rich source of information for comparisons and differences, enabling us to see what it is that human beings seem to require in order to develop a healthy interest in life – some mental and physical curiosity and vigour and pleasure in the world, rather than just the capacity to survive. Purely physical survival alone must almost always be questioned and emotional shutdown in a young baby should always give cause for concern.

In the close observation of infants we have the opportunity to see links between emotion and cognition; between feeling states in the mother and those in the infant; between the actual support available to a mother and her capacity in turn to support and encourage the physical, cognitive and emotional development of her child. We see the impact of unemployment, divorce, death of a family member, severe illness (in the infant or mother or other), migration, as well as other factors on a particular infant's development. Gradually patterns emerge; we can see some patterns repeated over and over again in similar but never identical circumstances.

Observing infants brings home the infinite variety in human life situations. There are so many variables – we may find two babies, observed in the same seminar, where both fathers become unemployed in the course of the observation. In the first family there may be considerable emotional and possibly financial support from other family members or friends. In the second family, by contrast, there may be no support of any kind forthcoming. What becomes apparent then is the *difference* between two families, each in stressful situations, caused by unemployment. It is therefore both the *similarities* and the *differences* in internal and external resources which become of equal relevance and interest and indicate important areas for research.

Over time, and with several infants observed (see Stephen Briggs, Chapter 12), patterns emerge which are common to all the infants, even where there are other variables. This understanding, real knowledge, is then available to inform social policy decisions. The discovery of similarities and differences makes for crude comparisons of little value if some cognisance is not taken of the details of the different circumstances of each family. Each infant observed can be taken as his or her own control in terms of research. Hypotheses can be made and tested throughout an observation. An infant can be followed up subsequently (see Gertraud Diem-Wille, Chapter 11) and the methodology described by Diem-Wille can be developed and adapted to follow up infants into adulthood.

Any teacher of infant observation will accumulate a vast 'resource' of infants observed for comparison. I am conscious of the richness of experience for myself; nothing else has afforded me the same opportunity for insight into human development; nothing else has made, and continues to make, me question every 'fact' I read about the development of our species. Nothing else informs and *changes* my clinical practice in the same way.

Every child psychotherapist, like every mental health professional and indeed every concerned adult, is preoccupied by the rise of violence and delinquency in ever younger children. The conditions for healthy versus unhealthy development are extremely complicated, and the interactions between the internal and the external worlds are profoundly complex. Nevertheless, the study of infancy provides an important searchlight on to the early origins of emotional disturbance. Where experiences in infancy have not promoted healthy emotional development, it becomes important to understand the impact of particular kinds of deprivation and/or abuse on subsequent character development.

The methodology used by Briggs in this book in exploring factors involved for 'at risk' infants paves the way for further important research with other categories of infants. This may shed light on the issue of what it is that is needed in order to ensure that the difficulties of one generation are minimised in the next.

The impact of intergenerational patterns of child-rearing are vividly revealed by observing infants, as this extract from an observation suggests:

Feeding Sally had never been enjoyable for either mother or baby. Other areas of their life were much more enjoyable for both of them. Sally was quickly switched from Mother's breast to the bottle, but bottle feeding became 'a job to be done' as quickly as possible. When Mum introduced solids to little Sally, the need, by mother, to control the feed became more and more apparent. The observer noted, feed after feed, the way in which mother firmly held on to bowl and spoon. Sally was never allowed to hold the spoon or touch her food, certainly not to play with it and explore its qualities. Mother made it clear that this feeding business was to be got through as quickly and cleanly as possible.

The observer found watching the feeds an extremely tense and uncomfortable business. With each spoonful the spoon was pushed far into baby's mouth, sometimes causing her to gag. Mother seemed not to notice this. After each mouthful mother stopped to scrape the spoon around the outside of Sally's mouth (like giving her a shave) to collect any bits that had escaped. This was then also quickly popped into Sally's mouth. The bowl was scraped clean and the last bit put into Sally. Mother never changed her rhythm, never checked to see Sally's response, never questioned whether she was enjoying her food, nor whether she wanted more or had had enough.

At six months this mother returned to work, leaving Sally in the care of her own mother during the day; she thoughtfully made arrangements for the observer to continue her observation of Sally in grandmother's home. The first observation in the new setting was duly brought to the seminar group. The shock was palpable. In the observation of the feed, Sally's grandmother fed her in an *identical* fashion to Sally's mother. It was like watching a mirror image. We could only conjecture that Sally's grandmother fed Sally's mother in just the same way that her mother had fed her. Of course, it was obvious that she would have no conscious memory of this, but perhaps an unconscious blueprint had been made of the experience. It seemed to have survived totally unmodified.

We questioned in our seminar group whether it had survived in this way, encapsulated, because mother, like Sally herself, had not found a way of protesting or resisting an obviously unsatisfactory and unpleasant experience. They had apparently been passive recipients. A link to the unmetabolised passing on of more major traumatic experiences, may be relevant. We can of course wonder how grandmother's mother in turn fed her. When did this particular pattern of feeding start? And, of course, why is there no apparent resistance – is there a genetic inheritance of passivity and/or is something else going on? We could not know the answers to these questions from one observation but it did raise questions and alert each of us to things we might previously have missed. That we inherit our parents' genes is undisputed; that we also inherit our parents' way of being, via their whole style of child-rearing is perhaps not so readily understood. (It should be emphasised here that this was a very 'ordinary' mother whose overall parenting was loving and caring.)

It becomes apparent from this, perhaps, that observing infants may also be an important source of information for the nature/nurture debate. Infant observation reveals just how complex and intertwined are the inherited disposition and the nurturing environment into which we are born. One constantly impacts upon the other. The work of Piontelli (1992), for example, pushes the debate back to the environment of the womb. Piontelli's fascinating research reveals just how ignorant we have been about life *in utero*. Her ultrasound studies of infants reveal that even identical twins, where they share the same placenta, do not experience identical conditions.

Many adults complain when they find themselves, as parents, sounding just like their own mother or father, especially when it is an aspect of that parent that they do not actually like or admire. It seems to have got right inside them and is hard to escape. It is very different, of course, to find oneself doing something in harmony with some appreciated quality in one's parents. No parent, of course, is perfect. Most parents try to do things for their baby, to the best of their ability, and often struggle to do better than they felt their own parents were able to do for them in certain areas. Sometimes patterns of parenting remain quite unconscious; when they are positive that is all well and good; when they are negative then there is cause for concern.

In the helping professions, or as researchers or academics, if we can learn from infant observation what makes for healthy development, then, as well as affecting our professional decisions, such observations can become a source of important information to be used in the critical examination of social policy. Our contributions, according to our professions, will be different, but can work in parallel.

CONCLUSION

I should perhaps add a final note: the method has been extended to the observation of young children and to a variety of work settings for more than twenty years. One extension is the observation of a group of elderly people in a residential home. They, like many of the observed families, showed considerable benefit from being the subjects of such close interest and attention. Experiences such as this have paved the way for the development of therapeutic infant observation.

The three parts of this book illustrate only a few of the exciting new developments in the practice of infant observation, in innovative contributions to theory and in qualitative research.

REFERENCES

Bick, E. (1964) 'Infant observation in psychoanalytic training', *International Journal of Psycho-Analysis*, 45: 558–566.

Bion, W. R. (1962) *Learning from Experience*, London: Heinemann.

Bion, W. R. (1965) *Transformations*, London: Heinemann.

Brazelton, T. B., Koslowski, B. and Main, M. (1974) 'The early mother–infant interaction', in M. Lewis and L. A. Rosenblum (eds) *The Effect of the Infant on its Caregivers*, London: Wiley Interscience.

Main, M. and Hesse, E. (1992) 'Disorganized/disoriented infant behaviour in the Strange Situation: lapses in the monitoring of reason and discourse during the parents' Adult Attachment Interview and dissociated states', in M. Ammaniti and D. Stern (eds) *Attachment and Psychoanalysis*, Rome: Gius, La Terza.

Miller, L., Rustin, M. E., Rustin, M. J. and Shuttleworth, J. (1989) *Closely Observed Infants*, London: Duckworth.

Piontelli, A. (1992) *From Foetus to Child: An Observational and Psychoanalytic Study*, London: Routledge.

Spitz, R. A. (1946) 'Anaclitic depression', *Psychoanalytic Study of the Child*, 2: 313–342.

Stern, D. (1985) *The Interpersonal World of the Infant*, New York: Basic Books.

Trevarthen, C. (1976) 'Descriptive analyses of infant communicative behavior', in H. R. Schaffer, (ed.) *Studies in Mother–Infant Interaction*, London: Academic Press.

Part I

The practice of infant observation

Introduction

Susan Reid

Part I of the book draws together those chapters which are primarily concerned with aspects of the actual practice of infant observation and the context within which these observations take place.

These chapters, taken together, make it clear that observing an infant in this way is not something undertaken lightly. The commitment from and to a particular family, together with the privilege of being allowed into such intimate contact with the emotional life of other human beings, finds a parallel only in clinical practice. It is one of the reasons why it is considered such a useful training experience for anyone intending to become a psychoanalytic psychotherapist, and why it has become valued by so many other professional trainings. The responsibility to the observed family and to the seminar group in the endeavour to make 'truthful' observations, sometimes in the face of considerable discomfort, is relived within these chapters.

In Chapter 2, 'Beginnings: the family, the observer and the infant observation group', Isca Wittenberg describes the experience of infant observation for the observer, seminar group and seminar leader, making links between the observer's experience and those of the infant. She vividly describes the intense primitive anxieties aroused by all 'beginnings'; the beginning of life for the infant, the beginning of an observation for the observer, and of a new observation group for the seminar leader. She parallels the needs of new infants in their families, if they are to develop and learn about the world around them, with the needs of new observers if they are to learn about the emotional life of the infant.

This chapter clearly elucidates the concept of 'containment' as used in psychoanalytic thinking: Wittenberg underlines the essential requirement for the seminar leader to 'hold' the anxieties of seminar members if they in turn are to be able to tolerate and 'contain' the disturbances evoked in them at infantile levels, through such intimate contact with the primitive anxieties observed in a baby.

Isca Wittenberg makes complex ideas and experiences accessible. She digs deeply into her own experiences to share the learning process honestly with the reader.

In Chapter 3, 'Shared unconscious and conscious perceptions in the nanny–parent interaction which affect the emotional development of the infant', Jeanne Magagna explores the role of the nanny (or other mother surrogate) as a significant attachment figure for the infant. She describes the social changes in the role of women in Western society which have led to many more infants being cared for by a mother surrogate in their formative years. She notes that mothers are the almost exclusive caregiver in only 3 per cent of societies in the world. Despite this, only a small number of psychoanalytic writings explore the psychological significance of the nanny or surrogate. She describes how an adult's inability to become involved in intimate relationships may be associated with the unmourned loss of a nanny in infancy.

The particular focus of the chapter is the concept of 'shared internal image', which is derived from Henry Dicks's (1967) concept, first used to describe unconscious phantasy systems extant between married couples. Here it is developed to explore the structure of the shared internal phantasy informing the relationship between the mother, nanny and baby. In the beginning is the parents' choice of a particular nanny and the nanny's choice to work for a particular family, then the ongoing interactions between mother (father)/nanny and baby; these may be more or less healthy, depending upon the nature of the shared internal image. Jeanne Magagna describes six shared internal images which she has encountered over her twenty-five years of observing infants and their families, using material drawn from infant observations to illustrate each example.

The ideas are linked to clinical practice, via a clinical example drawn from the work of Martha Harris. She underlines the importance of taking a careful history in any assessment if we are to uncover the possible role and influence of any mother surrogate.

This chapter pays due recognition to the reality that, in any seminar group today, several of the infants may be cared for by someone other than mother, for part of the time. This is a radical and rapid change in Great Britain, occurring over the last twenty-five years. This change has had a significant impact on family life as most of the parents we observe have been looked after exclusively by their parents. They are, however, in the position of leaving their own infant in the care of someone else, usually because both parents are working. Where there is no tradition of this, the parents are entering new territory which can cause extreme anxiety. Amongst the enormous database of observed infants collected over the years, we therefore have the possibility for some more formal research, comparing those babies cared for exclusively by their parents with those where surrogate care has been used. (See Part III, on research developments.)

In Chapter 4, 'The meaning of difference: race, culture and context in infant observation', Lynda Ellis focuses on how socio-cultural constructions shape and influence what we see as observers, highlighting the potential for significant aspects of the observation to be lost, misunderstood or distorted. This chapter focuses upon an area in infant observation which has previously been neglected in the literature, but which has increasing relevance in the multi-racial, multi-cultural societies in which many of us now live.

Observations of infants from a range of cultural and racial backgrounds open up an area of enormous potential richness in exploring issues of similarity and difference, providing due attention is paid to the concerns Lynda Ellis raises in terms of cross-cultural bias, when the infant observed is from a different cultural, racial or class background to the observer.

With a background in sociology, Ellis is moving into unfamiliar territory, from the culture of 'environment' to the culture of psychoanalysis, 'the internal world'. This parallels the situation of the observed family, who are also struggling to find a place. The honesty with which this struggle is charted, together with the vivid observational material, allows the reader to share both experiences. Ellis recognises that she missed the significance to the family of a visitor from their home country; the anxiety not to stereotype can actually interfere with the capacity to see what is really there.

Ellis shares with the reader the painful but enriching process of becoming an observer. This complements Isca Wittenberg's chapter on 'Beginnings' – exploring, along with the significance of 'difference', the impact of 'beginning' something new for *one* observer and *one* family.

It is in the synthesis of the two cultures of sociology and psychoanalysis that something new emerges; a contribution to psychoanalytic thinking and to sociology.

This chapter illustrates the impact on the emotional and cognitive development of an infant when his family is uprooted from the familiar culture which provides 'containment' for the parents to one where familiarity is lost; it is replaced by an alien, often unfriendly and unwelcoming culture where the parents' adult capacities are undermined. Lynda Ellis's chapter is helpful to an understanding that an approach to mothering which has developed in one particular cultural context may be at odds with the expectations and infrastructure of a different socio-cultural environment, and may consequently put the infant at risk.

The potential for exploring, via this close observational method, what is held in common by all human infants and what is environmentally influenced, is truly exciting.

In this way, Chapter 4 links with Chapter 2 on 'Beginnings' in showing how, to some degree, both becoming an observer and becoming parents are potentially overwhelming experiences because they take us into unfamiliar territory – just as choosing a nanny for those who have never had one, have not had the *experience* of being nannied, is also potentially overwhelming. Another thread which draws these three chapters together, then, is the understanding that overwhelming anxiety, when it cannot be contained by ourselves or another, threatens our capacity to think and feel, and therefore undermines our capacity to make thoughtful decisions.

The observational method, illuminated by these chapters, underlines the importance of recognising the contribution in *all* father–mother–infant relationships of the internal worlds of the parents, the character of the infant, and the environment in which they live.

REFERENCE

Dicks, H. (1967) *Marital Tensions*, London: Routledge and Kegan Paul.

Chapter 2

Beginnings
The family, the observer and the infant observation group

Isca Wittenberg

INTRODUCTION

In this chapter, I set out to show some of the linked and parallel processes which take place within a group studying infant observation and those which occur in the families observed.

When I began to think about my conference paper and decided to speak about beginnings, I promptly had a nightmare. I shall recount it briefly because I consider it to be a social dream in the sense that Gordon Lawrence (Lawrence 1991) speaks of social dreaming as embodying the preoccupations of a group, rather than expressing merely the personal concerns of the dreamer. The dream illustrates the fears, conscious and unconscious, which are aroused whenever we face new experiences, new beginnings.

The dream

In my dream, I had driven a group to a little town where we were to explore old buildings and new developments. After we had walked together for some time, I got separated from the rest of the group. Although somewhat disturbed by this, I became seriously alarmed when I realised that we would need to meet up again before we could proceed to the next city or indeed go back to the one we had come from, as there was no other means of transport but this car. It occurred to me then that the obvious thing was to make my way back to where the car had been parked, and I expected the rest of the group to do the same. But, when I got to that place, the others were not to be seen, nor was the car. I then remembered, to my great consternation, that I had moved the car from the original parking spot because of the amount of heavy traffic passing by. How now would the others find the car and find me? I asked some shoppers whether they had seen the group, but they had not. It occurred to me that I might get some help at the police station, but when I asked the way, I was warned that this would mean passing through some dangerous areas. Suddenly, I found I could neither remember the street I had left the car in, nor the name of the place which we had originally come from that morning. I woke up in a panic.

When I began to think about the dream, I became aware that I had once again experienced fears of beginning something new; namely, feeling alone, lost, separated and disconnected from familiar places, the familiar group, afraid of dangers. Furthermore, there was the fear of not finding the way back to a haven of safety. It is what Dr Bion (Bion 1966) called 'catastrophic anxiety', our terror which is linked to the tremendous and terrifying change at the caesura of birth. Such deep-seated anxiety connected with any change inclines us to cling to the familiar throughout life. We are terrified of feeling disconnected from the externally known and unconnected to our precarious inner orientation and in-touchness. It threatens whenever we go into physical, mental or emotional new territory and yet, as Bion showed, it is the capacity to face such anxieties and take risks which is essential for mental and/or emotional growth to take place. Otherwise, we are precluded from finding out, from getting to know, from having any truly new experience. The dream also showed me that in anticipating the conference, far from feeling that we were all following along the same path, as I had originally imagined, I was secretly afraid that this group, brought together by the shared training in and passion for infant observation, might have gone so much their separate ways that we might not find each other again, or that one would be abandoned by the group if one had moved away from the original 'parking place', i.e., the shared way of thinking and acting. Both these possibilities seemed to preclude the meeting of minds from which we could move forward together.

I would like to turn now to my own beginnings in infant observation. I had the good fortune to have Dr Esther Bick, the originator of the infant observation groups, as my teacher. She had a great capacity to be in touch with and convey the baby's experience: the desperate means which the baby adopts in his fight for survival; the bringing together of the infant's self around the sensation of nipple-in-mouth; the mother's holding of the baby's disparate parts thus providing a physical/mental/emotional skin, essential as a basis for healthy development. All this, as well as the defensive measures the baby adopts when the mother is unable to provide this holding, was not only an inspiration at the time but over the years has become ever more meaningful to me. Equally, her awareness of the new parents' persecutory and depressive anxieties and hence the great care the observer needs to take not to exacerbate these, has left a deep mark.

In a way, of course, infant observation, though a convenient term, is a misnomer, for we do not only observe the baby. In fact what we study is the nature of an interaction, the link between baby and the world, the world which at first is primarily conveyed through the mother. This link between mother and baby is so close, so intimately interactive, that Middlemore (1941) called this twosome 'the nursing couple'. Of course this does not mean that one does not pay the greatest attention to the infant's feelings and behaviour. It is, however, important that at the preliminary meeting students express their interest in learning how a baby develops relationships. If they merely state that they want to observe a baby, this may lead to misunderstanding and they may find themselves left looking after the child while mother busies herself around the house. I have known this happen to observers partly because, at the initial interview, they had stated that they wanted to observe a baby rather than saying that they were interested to learn how a baby forms relationships. It no longer seems accurate to say that we observe the baby from the very beginning of life. The infant, at entry into the external world, brings not only a genetic endowment, but the history of intra-uterine life as well as the birth experience, all of which together help to predispose the baby to certain expectations about life outside. Mother and father come to the event of the baby's birth with a history of their external and internal worlds.

Equally, in a seminar, an interactive process between members of the group develops, partly based on their experience of the present and, in addition, on what they bring with them in terms of their own personal history, their preconceptions and their theoretical frameworks.

THE PREGNANCY STAGE

At the beginning of the academic year, I am, like most teachers of infant observation, in an expectant state wondering what the new baby-observation group soon due to begin will be like. I hope and pray that I will have students who come with good endowment and potential for emotional growth and development. I used to be anxious about whether there would be enough for us to discuss if students had not found babies by the time the teaching term started. Such anxiety communicates itself to students, who in turn become anxious whether any family will have them and hence whether they will have a baby in time. I think this was borne out at a review meeting when a student said: 'It would be helpful if we were told that it is a two-year seminar, but we do not need to have a baby right away.' The 'pregnancy' stage of the group seems to me now so important that I encourage students to do no more beforehand than think about whom they might contact in order to find a family during the first term. In order for students to get the most out of the opportunity to observe, they need a holding environment and quite especially so at the very beginning. We may know about the baby's need for holding, feeding, evacuation, for the conversion of sense data into meaning: we may believe that mothers need containing so that they can cope with the anxieties of pregnancy, of giving birth and the first few months of the baby's life. We may not, however, always give enough consideration to the students' need for containment as they begin to observe a family and become involved in seeing a highly emotionally charged drama unfold before their eyes. They too are entering a new world, born as students into a new course of study, feeling lost in new surroundings, a new group, a new teacher and, especially, a new way of looking at human relationships.

When students have plunged into observing without careful preparation, it has usually been because they were beset by worries about whether they would ever succeed in finding a baby to observe. One student feared that, as a man, he stood little chance of doing so, and when he was offered a family with a 5-week-old infant, he jumped at the opportunity. It was sad, and now he thinks so too, that he was not in on the first few weeks of the baby's life, so vital for development. It is true of course, that in any case we see only a fraction of the myriad happenings and changes that the baby undergoes, but not to observe in the early weeks when the most primitive anxieties and ways of dealing with them are foremost and can be studied, seems to me not only to miss the very basis of understanding that baby's development but to miss learning from the experience of being a participant observer, about the very depth of very powerful infantile anxieties. The student also missed the opportunity to hear about foetal behaviour and the parents' phantasies about the unborn infant. He did not have the chance to get an impression of the parents as a couple, and their home as indicative of their inner world before the baby was born.

Another student, on her own initiative, went to a Maternity and Child Welfare Centre where she was introduced to a mother-to-be who on the spot agreed to the Health Visitor's suggestion that her baby be observed. Perhaps it is not surprising to learn that this arrangement, so casually entered into, soon broke down. At the second visit, the observer found the door barred and, on telephoning, was informed by the father that his wife was too depressed and harassed to want to see her then, or at any later point. The student in turn became depressed, feeling a failure because of this abortive beginning.

The expectancy stage for the student, when they do not know whether there will be a viable baby to observe, mirrors the parents' doubts before and during pregnancy, and thus helps us to be in touch with these doubts. Empathic understanding of the parents' anxieties about the firstborn might be helped by a perusal of Christopher Clulow's book, *To Have and to Hold* (1982) and by reading reports of interviews with parents of infants seen in the Under-Fives Counselling Service in the Child and Family Department at the Tavistock Clinic (Wittenberg 1991: 83–105).

It seems essential to allow plenty of time within the seminar group for other preparatory discussions. What might be said to those professionals who might put the student in touch with expectant parents? We need to allow students to air their doubts about entering a family as an observer; for example, whether it is justifiable to use observations of such intimate relationships for one's professional training. Much time needs to be spent discussing the student's role in the family: how one can be a listener and observer, an interested person who is neither a friend nor an advice-giver, nor behaves like a piece of wood.

Where there are second-year students in the group, they can tell the newcomers of their experiences far better and from a closer range than the seminar leader. The first observation group I started, in Oslo in 1977, consisting mainly of staff members of the Mentalhygiensk Clinic, decided to role-play the preliminary visit to parents. The feedback of what it felt like to be 'the mother', 'the father' and 'the observer' proved to be both fun and very helpful.

BIRTH: THE NEED TO HOLD THE BABY AND THE GROUP

Whatever the preparation, the actual birth of a baby is a momentous event, a matter of life and death, of terror and fulfilment, of relief and joy. Nothing will ever be the same as it was before for any member of the family. The baby is exposed to a totally unfamiliar environment: limited, bounded space being replaced by boundaryless-ness; connectedness to life-sustaining supplies replaced by separateness from the source of food, warmth and safety, and the infant's senses bombarded by powerful, sensual impressions. The infant has lost all it knows through the caesura of birth and may temporarily lose some of the capacities previously developed *in utero*.

Our students also lose and need to lose some of what is part of their internal equipment, namely, their assumptions about babyhood, their educational principles, their moral evaluation of parenthood and their use of theories as armoury to hold themselves together, rather than being open to new, disturbing experiences. Just as the baby and his parents are finding out about each other with a sense of alert and deep interest (if they are not too overwhelmed by what they see, hear, smell and feel), so one hopes that students can maintain their curiosity and in-touchness in spite of, or because of, the powerful emotions stirred up by the experience.

Students often express their not inappropriate fear of intruding on the family, but what they may be less aware of is their fear of being intruded upon, invaded by the impact of what they are observing, receiving and having to contain. Being born into the role of observer is invariably traumatic because we have all defended against deep infantile anxieties by idealising babies and babyhood. To actually witness the baby's frequent falling apart, to become aware of how little we know of what the baby wants at times when it cannot be comforted, to observe what agonies babies, mothers and fathers go through, is always a shocking discovery for the inexperienced observer.

One student who began her observations during the Christmas break told us months afterwards that she had found the first few weeks totally overwhelming and could barely stay out the hour. This was, in fact, not a particularly disturbed relationship, just an ordinary mother and baby. In addition, she felt angry at not having been able to bring her observations to the group until term started. Her scanty, vague notes certainly indicated that she had not been able to take in much. It had been too painful to see, so she, like all of us when we are overwhelmed emotionally, turned a blind eye. For this reason, it is helpful, as far as possible, to stagger the beginning of observations, to create a space for each student to present the baby after the first or second post-natal visit.

The discussion by the group helps to sort out different elements, to get hold of the experience, to begin to get a picture of this particular baby and, while we are aware that these are only first impressions, they are nevertheless highly significant. They provide a basis from which some orientation, some searching for meaning, and many questions about further details to be looked for, emerge. Sometimes it opens the observer's eyes to far more pain than they had been aware of and wish to be in touch with, but mostly such group discussions help the observer to feel that they, and the family, are held by the group's concern. It was particularly useful for a group from abroad to discuss one baby for most of one weekend. This detailed study helped the whole group to begin to appreciate how much there is to see, wonder and think about in our attempt to arrive at some meaningful picture of each unique mother/father/baby triad.

The survival of a whole seminar group can be threatened if it is not sufficiently held at the beginning. This was brought home to me when asked to help a newly formed infant observation group in Eastern Europe. I decided to go there only when two or more members of the group had already begun observing. I rationalised this decision on the basis that there were two psychoanalysts in the group who had attended infant observation seminars at the Tavistock. I thought they could prepare the group by relating their experiences, as well as reading Mrs Bick's paper (Bick 1964: 558–566), Jeanne Magagna's description of seminars with Mrs Bick (Magagna 1987: 19–41) and the book, *Closely Observed Infants* (Miller *et al.* 1989). I failed to take into consideration that this group was not part of an institution nor part of a more extensive course.

On my first visit I found a very disparate group. The two analysts were highly committed and were in fact carrying the whole burden of organisation, including being the only ones prepared to take notes of the group discussions. Of the remaining three, one man seemed very interested but highly intellectually defended; he also made it clear that he would not be able to start observing for another nine months. One woman – Mrs A

– doubted whether family commitments would permit her to continue and the fifth member – Mr F – had seen the mother and baby a few times and found it extremely disturbing. It wasn't a 'cosy' experience; I am sure he had not been led to believe that observing an infant would be cosy, but he was clearly not inwardly prepared for how frightening he would find the actual experience.

It was in fact a disturbing situation with a mother who was unable to hold the baby close and was extremely controlling with him. She had yielded to her husband's wish for a baby by becoming pregnant soon after marriage, but he was working long hours and therefore not able to give much support to his wife. Mother longed to go back to work and did so after a very short time. Moreover, the au pair girl was instructed not to allow the baby to comfort himself by sucking his thumb and she stuck to this most of the time, in spite of the baby's distress. She also often stopped him, as the mother had done, reaching out for objects that interested him.

It seemed when discussing the material that the observer was very much in touch with the baby's suffering but so agonised by it that he recoiled from what he saw and felt. In the ensuing weeks, he retreated to a tough attitude, which allowed him to hold on to the belief that the baby's great distress and the constant rigid holding of his arms at right angles to his body, was quite ordinary, nothing to be concerned about. By the time of my second visit, six weeks later, Mrs A said that she wanted to stop and Mr F had definitely decided to discontinue the observations, saying he was too busy. In vain did we try to convince him that when he had visited he had acted as someone who contained some of the anxiety of the baby and the au pair girl, who in fact seemed somewhat more relaxed now in her handling of the baby. We pointed out that the baby would experience yet another loss and expressed our worry that his leaving would further undermine the mother's belief in the baby's goodness as well as in her maternal capacities. The heated discussion went on for a very long time but Mr F was adamant. Eventually, we managed to persuade him to continue at least for another two months on a less frequent basis, and to discuss with the mother how she felt about this. I was very shocked at Mr F's irresponsibility in just dropping the family, and the lack of insight shown by maintaining that his leaving did not matter in the least as there was no alive relationship. To our horror, he was so out of touch that he suggested that, if we felt so strongly, then he could just send a student of his to take his place as an observer in the family. But most of all, I held myself responsible for not sufficiently taking care of the beginning of this group, and thus not providing an emotional environment which held the members.

It also became clear that weekend that the whole of this infant observation group's life was at stake, for with two people dropping out and another due to move to London in a few months' time, it would no longer be financially viable. Fighting for the survival of Mr F's baby observation and of this group evoked in me memories of the death and destruction of families in Nazi times, and I worked at such fever pitch to try and save the situation that in the end I became acutely ill. Such is the powerful impact of baby observation and of a group! We cannot, must not, treat it lightly. It is the opportunity to go back to the beginning of life that makes infant observation so worthwhile, stimulating us to get in touch with our own primitive anxieties, holding both terror and great potential for thought and emotional development.

As leaders of infant observation groups, we are doubly privileged, for, in addition to studying development *in statu nascendi*, we are privy to our students' discovery of infantile life and the rediscovery of the infant part of the self. While this is, in the true sense of the word, wonderful, it is also awesome, for it places a great responsibility on our shoulders both to the families observed and to our students in helping them to hold the anxieties they go through in the course of this experience. Like a good parent, the teacher needs to provide an environment which modulates persecutory and depressive anxiety so that making links is not too frightening, so that one dares to dream, phantasise, discover reality, feel feelings, think thoughts in spite of the feared destructiveness from outside and within.

Luckily, some babies survive inadequate mothering, and so it was with some members of this group. They were determined to go on, found others interested to join and were eager for these participants to come in right away; but I insisted that this time we would begin slowly and carefully, and that prospective members should just sit in and listen before they made a decision to join. On the basis of our experience, the structure of the course, the commitment in terms of time and finance, of frequency of meetings, with and without a teacher from London, were all thoroughly discussed and agreed. Out of these troubled beginnings grew a hard-working, closely knit infant observation group.

ESTABLISHING FEEDING, PLAYING AND A WORKING RELATIONSHIP

Like the mother who is not sure whether her breast will be able to produce milk, whether there is enough milk and whether it is sufficiently nourishing for the baby, I am often worried during seminars that I may have nothing to say, afraid that I will not be able to make sense of what I hear and that my contribution will not be good enough. Afterwards, however, I often fear that I have been over-feeding the group, speaking too much by responding spontaneously to the material presented, voicing whatever thoughts and feelings it has evoked in me. I do not want members to be adhesive to my feeding, but to think for themselves. I encourage members of the group to give free rein to their associations around what they have heard. I find it helpful for us to enact the baby's movements, vocal and facial expressions, and in this way to try to get inside the baby's sensuous, emotional experience via our own bodies; to see what it feels like and what it might mean. I think of this freedom to experiment and phantasise in terms of what Winnicott called the 'play-area' (Winnicott 1971), a space for creative thought belonging neither wholly to the object or the subject but arising from their relatedness.

But then we need to ask ourselves 'Where's the evidence?' for our assumptions. I find that students appreciate that free-ranging thoughts are useful yet should not be allowed simply to stand unchallenged. They are firmly led back to the details of the observation and the context in which a piece of behaviour occurred to see whether our ideas fit or not and later check this also against subsequent observations. Sometimes, I find it helps to make links to what members of the group are more familiar with, i.e., manifestations in childhood and adolescence of, for instance, pseudo-independence, eating disorders and other kinds of somatic symptoms as well as autistic features. At times, the material and our exchanges stimulate us to make new discoveries, or rather see what in a way is obvious; for instance, suddenly being struck, in the course of an observation of a baby who had spent a month in an incubator and continued to prefer the bottle to breast, that it was the bottle which had been his first contact with mother, his first feeding object and that he had been, so to speak, 'weaned' from the bottle onto the breast.

In her paper, 'Notes on infant observation in psychoanalytic training', Esther Bick (1964) takes a rather kindly view of the critical attitude towards mothers that so commonly besets observers. She considers it to be the result of the mother's projection of her self-doubts and depression into the observer. That may well be so, but envy of parents and competition with them may also be at work. I have come to think that there is another very important factor involved in the attractiveness of blaming parents and speculating about them endlessly. It is clear that at times it is a flight reaction, either a flight from the observer's experience of not knowing and the catastrophic anxiety aroused by this, or a flight from finding what is seen to be unbearably painful. In these circumstances comments tend to shift away from the baby to a demonisation of the parents and an implied idealisation of the baby. When observers become persecuted by the anxieties picked up in the observation, then there is a danger that they, in their own minds, start persecuting the parents. Perhaps all of us have a wish to hold on to the idea of a Messiah baby, who represents our wish for total goodness and hope for the future. I believe that persecutory and depressive anxieties of parents and observers alike come to the fore when they realise that this is not the case. It is a shockingly disappointing experience to face the fact that babies, as well as being lovely, wonderful, full of potential, are also demanding, possessive and can be cruel, biting, envious and ungrateful; others may be lacking in life-force or the desire to make constructive links with the world. When we become aware of such disturbing aspects we tend to prefer to put any difficulty the baby manifests down to the parent's inadequacies.

HOLDING ANGER, DESPAIR AND HOPE

In any seminar, situations are likely to arise which are especially difficult to bear. Just as the parents' function is to go on puzzling, thinking, staying with the pain and still go on hoping, so one finds that one has to hold on to and convey to the group a hope that there might be some way in which the situation might improve, might be bearable, might be capable of change. At least we can attempt to understand it even if we can do little to change it.

Miss W's first impression when she visited the home of the family she had come to observe was of a subdued, controlled atmosphere. Mother appeared absent-minded and the two older children played away from mother but were keen to involve the observer. The baby was kept much of the time out of sight, his pram tucked away behind a filing cabinet. Mother attended to him only when she thought he needed feeding or changing. She was gentle in her handling but there seemed to be no real emotional involvement. The baby did not look at his mother, but he fed well and he did not cry when the breast was removed, indeed he hardly ever showed any distress. Most of the time he lay in his pram, curled up and quite still. The members of the seminar found it difficult to hold on to Ivor, as I shall call him. We could not visualise him as a person and we could not remember him from one presentation to the next. We became aware that this was a repetition of the baby's experience within his family as a forgotten, dropped-out-of-mind baby.

Every time the observer visited the home, she expected the mother would tell her not to come any more. She became worried also about not being a good-enough student. As she expressed it later:

> I was afraid I was not giving the right material to the group, was not seeing what emotional interaction was in fact happening, wondered whether I was only able to dwell on a description of the older children's behaviour because I was not in touch with the infant.

It was possible for us to convey to her that she was holding and expressing the baby's feelings of having nothing to offer the mother that might interest or enliven her. An adult patient put it this way: 'I was not able to put the roses back into my mother's cheeks.' Miss W said later:

> At an intuitive level I knew there was something wrong in the family

but I was not able to process what was happening. I felt something was hidden, just like the baby who himself seemed to hide his distress, being no problem.

In the fourth month, the observer was tempted to terminate the observations. She says:

> I had stuck with the family hoping things would improve, but it became too difficult. I felt excluded and unwanted. I could not see much of the baby and at the same time felt I could not make any further demands on this depressed mother. I became invaded by hopelessness and dread as if something very terrifying was being hidden. For a couple of weeks, the observations were so painful that I was unable to write them up, which compounded my feelings of being no good as an observer.

We sympathised with the observer's despair and took it as her identification with the baby and perhaps also with the mother. We encouraged her to continue observing, pointing out that she seemed to provide some containment for the mother and children, some point of hope, and that to give up would confirm the mother's and children's belief in not being worthwhile staying with. And then, one day, the mother knocked on the observer's door and poured out her heart, talking very openly about the crisis in her marriage which had been going on since before Ivor's birth. At this point the mother had decided not simply to put up with her husband's secret affair but to make a stand. With this, the atmosphere of an impending hidden disaster and the projection into the observer of feeling unwanted faded. As a result the observations were less dreaded, although the pain and worry about Ivor's development remained.

In a second, very different example, a student described the parental couple he observed as being cold and aloof and the little baby girl from the beginning appeared very lifeless. Her arms and legs hung limply, she seemed like a puppet whose extremities had not yet been pulled together by connecting strings. The observer's presentations were equally lifeless and disjointed and so was the group as they listened to him. There seemed to be an atmosphere of resignation, if not boredom in the group. I found myself getting more and more frustrated and angry because I could not get a spark out of the student; there was very little response to my questions and comments. Eventually, I put into words what I felt, saying that I wondered whether perhaps he felt equally angry and frustrated at having been landed with such a very difficult mother and baby. As a result of this intervention he came more alive and suddenly the mother seemed somewhat less lacking in personality and the whole situation capable of interested exploration.

In such situations the verbalisation of the leader's or the group's counter-transference feelings can be very helpful in restoring hope to the group and thus enable us to go on struggling to understand rather than giving up. The mere voicing of difficulties may be enough in itself: in one seminar group I expressed feeling worried and guilty that there never seemed enough time to do justice to the discussion of the twin babies being observed by one of the members. This not only corresponded to what it was like for the mother to have two little ones and never enough space, time and energy to attend adequately to both of them, but also to how the observer felt in trying to observe and record the observation of two babies and present them in the group. Similarly, when it has been acknowledged that it might be difficult for newcomers joining an established group, this has been appreciated. It has opened the way to their expressing their fear that they would never be able to bring as good observations, nor understand as much as the older members of the group; also the latter have been able to voice their resentment at new people coming into the group.

All these matters – holding, feeding, maintaining hope – become more complex when teaching takes place at less frequent intervals, as it does when teaching abroad. It is not enough to set up a structure. The beginnings are crucial; one needs to be more available, more frequently present until such time as a good working relationship has been established. The lack of containment, the infrequent feeding, the absence of firm leadership, all make it harder for a group to stick to the detail, to be in touch with primitive anxieties, to maintain hope, to refrain from escaping into preoccupation with the parents, from relying on theory and coming to premature omniscient conclusions. As a leader, one also faces additional problems. Sometimes it is harder to keep the babies alive in my mind and always I fear that I over-feed because of the shortage of time, that I do not give enough space to what I have called the play-area nor hear enough about the work that the group has done without me. There are, however, some precious qualities attached to these infrequent but long meetings. Not only does it make comparison between the different babies easier when they are presented one after the other, but spending a whole weekend studying babies makes for a very intense, very powerful and often deeply moving experience. While the long breaks make leave-taking more painful, the intense experience enables us to maintain a deep relationship over time and to await the next meeting eagerly.

ENDING AND BEGINNING AGAIN

Finally, I want to describe a meeting towards the end of the course with the group whose difficult starting phase I discussed earlier. It seemed as if in some ways we were back at the beginning. Our very intellectual member, who had much softened over the year and was deeply emotionally engaged, suddenly accused me of 'talking theory'; the rest of the group had difficulty in relating to the material and found what I said strange.

All this happened during a discussion of observations of the oldest baby in the group, then aged 16 months, whose mother was pregnant.

When the observer arrived, the little girl had been lying between two cushions in the parents' bed, and had wanted father to join her there, which he did. The observer had noticed that the child looked at her with a shy and anxious expression, although at all other times she had welcomed the observer with friendly smiles. I remarked on the little girl wanting to take mother's place and make babies with her father, an idea which seemed very much supported by her having later on brought a banana and yoghurt for her father to eat, dancing in front of him, and feeding her soft rabbit as if it was a baby. I remarked: 'No wonder she was wary of the observer seeing all this.' 'Really', someone said, 'Surely not. Anyway the observer is not the mother.' Eventually, I found myself exclaiming, 'How would you feel if you had an affair and a friend of the family discovered you both lying in bed. And what do you think about the plant the child was pulling out from underneath the table? Might this not be seen as her trying to get rid of the mother's inside baby?' I became more and more puzzled by the group's apparent inability to see the obvious, until it occurred to me that it was exactly a year since most of them had joined the group; that perhaps their unusual lack of perceptiveness might be due to the observation having evoked their own child-like feelings and fear that there would soon be a new baby-group to replace theirs. I suggested that they might like to think whether this was possibly something that got in the way today. The group came back next day, not referring directly to what I had said, but telling me that they had discussed their future.

They wanted to continue with the infant observation group and our meetings; not for another four months, as planned, or six months, but at least for a year and, when that finished, they wanted to go on to do child observation and after that a year's theory . . .

Sooner or later they will have to face the end of their observations, of the group and our seminars, of the relationship with their observed infants and their mothers and fathers, and their infant observation teachers. Like any ending, whether it be the end of pregnancy, of intra-uterine life, the end of babyhood, or childhood, so the end of an observation group means having to face all over again the anxieties of beginning. At the end, which spells a new beginning, what is re-evoked is helplessness in the face of the unknown, and the dread of having to survive separate from those we have come to rely on, fearing that we have not enough inner equipment to carry on by ourselves. Even if we do, we or others might destroy it. Yet in order to go forward we have to maintain hope in the goodness of our roots and gather our courage to extend from the more intimate connectedness, to making wider connections, and through imaginative leaps linking to the endless manifestations of life and mystery all around us in the world, well beyond our own little selves. Putting it in musical terms, there is a chain of connectedness from the sounds we perceive *in utero*, to the attachment to mother's voice and through that to an appreciation of the music of great composers, to the sounds in nature, the music of the spheres.

REFERENCES

Bick, E. (1964) 'Notes on infant observation in psychoanalytic training,' *International Journal of Psycho-Analysis*, 45: 558–566.

Bion, W. (1966) 'Catastrophic change', paper given to British Psycho-Analytic Society, in *British Psycho-Analytic Society and Institute of Psycho-Analysis Scientific Bulletin*, 5: 13–25.

Clulow, C. (1982) *To Have and to Hold: Marriage, the First Baby and Preparing Couples for Parenthood*, Aberdeen: Aberdeen University Press.

Lawrence, G. (1991) 'One from the void and formless infinite: experiences in social dreaming', *Free Association*, 2, 2: 259–294.

Magagna, J. (1987) 'Three years of infant observation with Mrs Bick', *Journal of Child Psychotherapy*, 13, 1: 19–41.

Middlemore, P. M. (1941) *The Nursing Couple*, London: Cassell.

Miller, L., Rustin, M. E., Rustin, M. J. and Shuttleworth, J. (eds) (1989) *Closely Observed Infants*, London: Duckworth.

Winnicott, D. (1971) *Playing and Reality*, London: Tavistock.

Wittenberg, I. (1991) 'Brief therapeutic work with parents of infants', in R. Szur and S. Miller (eds) *Extending Horizons*, London: Karnac.

Chapter 3

Shared unconscious and conscious perceptions in the nanny–parent interaction which affect the emotional development of the infant

Jeanne Magagna

The presence of a nanny plays a crucial role in the developing personality of the infant. The nanny being a significant attachment figure for the infant elicits a relationship with the infant which is unique and distinct from that which the infant has with the mother and the father. For this reason the role of nanny cannot be ignored. In this chapter I shall explore how the mother and nanny's unconsciously shared internal images can positively and negatively influence the infant's introjection of 'a good mother' which is the basis of healthy psychological development.

As there is considerable social change in the role of women, many more women are working outside the home. In fact, one-fifth of Britain's children spend their formative years in the care of 'surrogate mothers' while their mothers work. Mothers currently are the almost exclusive caregiver in only 3 per cent of societies in the world and the predominant caregivers in only 60 per cent of societies (Weisner and Gallimore 1977: 169–190).

Despite these facts, it is striking to find only a small number of psychoanalytic writings tracing the psychological significance of the nanny. When the infant has not been able to adequately mourn the absences or departures of the nanny, an aura of estrangement and loss can surround the child into adulthood. A person's inability to become involved in intimate relationships may be associated with the loss of a nanny. In therapy, the image of the mother may serve to function as a screen for the surrogate mother. For this reason, it is essential to note the presence of the substitute caregivers in the life of the child (Hardin 1985: 609–624).

Certainly the role of the nanny is prominent in the descriptions of lives of many famous people such as psychoanalysts Sigmund Freud and Melanie Klein, statesman Winston Churchill and writers Honoré de Balzac, Vladimir Nabokov, Antonia Fraser and Robert Louis Stevenson, to name but a few. Freud, for example, described his relationship with his nanny, saying: 'She provided me at such an early age with the means for living and surviving' (Freud 1954: 219–220). He suddenly lost her at the age of 2 , and in his self-analysis, Freud could not re-experience either the intensity or the exclusiveness of his tie with his nanny, nor did he experience the anguish following its severance. It seems that he was unable to bridge the gap between his mother and his nurse (Hardin 1986: 72–86).

Sachs (1971: 469–480) described how the inability to bear the loss of a nanny had been a major factor influencing the neurotic symptomatology of five of the six patients whose history she explored. For each patient, the departure of the nanny had a great impact during childhood. Sachs also described how the use of the nanny served various useful purposes. In particular she detailed how the nanny became a helpful receptacle for aggression in several children. The non-punitive, accepting attitude of the nanny enabled the child to feel it was possible to redirect sadistic impulses to the nanny which had been previously directed towards themselves. In another child the mother's harsh punitive behaviour towards the child's Oedipal jealousy and anger increased the severe persecutory guilt in the child. The nanny's presence was felt to be of great therapeutic importance for the child.

Meltzer (1994) describes a crucial task of development in the child which can be evaded through flight to an Oedipal entanglement with the nanny. He describes how, in order to introject mother, the child must tolerate the pain of giving the mother her freedom to come and go at will and suffer the burden of mother having a relationship with the siblings and the father. In a detailed study he shows how a child can develop a more prolonged, sensual, possessive and exclusive relationship with his nanny. In this way the child may blind himself to the beauty of his relationship with the mother and the pain of separation from her. Such an evasion of appreciation of the mother and painful conflict with her can interfere with the developmental task of integrating loving and hostile feelings towards her. Descriptions of the nanny's important influence on the child's developing personality have also been chronicled by other psychoanalysts including Fenichel (1954: 185), Winnicott (1976: 143), Deutsch (1963: 164), A. Freud (1946: 64) and Hardin (1985: 609–629).

Twenty-five years of observations of infants in their families and discussion groups with nannies leads me to conceive of the infant's 'family' as consisting not only of the mother, father and siblings, but also the 'nanny' or assistant caregivers, if present in the family's life-history. I am writing with a fundamental belief in the primary importance of the infant's relationship with the mother and an appreciation of the uniqueness of the infant's relationship with each caregiver. With these underlying assumptions present in my work, I shall show how the personality structure of the infant is influenced by the internalisation of the 'shared unconscious internal images' structuring the process of caregiving provided by the mother and nanny.

SHARED INTERNAL IMAGE

From infancy onwards each person has an unconscious inner world of figures formed on the pattern of the persons first loved and hated in life. The various parts of the self have relationships with these internal figures which also contain aspects of infantile phantasies and projections. There is a continuous but fluctuating unconscious internal drama of complex interactions of the internal figures. This unconscious internal drama both informs and is informed by the person's relationships in his external world. The pattern of unconscious relations between the internal parents and the infant part of the self influence a couple's choice of a nanny and the nanny's decision to work with a particular family. As the interaction between the nanny, the parents and the baby evolves, there is an interplay between the external activities and unconscious dramas existing within this 'family group'. From moment to moment and during certain stages in the lives of the infant and parents, there are fluctuations in the pattern of internal dramas and shared internal images.

The notion of the shared internal image is derived from Henry Dicks's (1967: 78, 79) concept described in his book *Marital Tensions*. The shared internal objects with their unconscious phantasy system colour the way in which partners give meaning to their social and intimate relationships and perform their roles. For example, one partner in the marriage could be carrying or acting as the container of aspects of the other's internal object relationships which the other cannot contain. One such situation would be when a woman unconsciously marries her 'idealised father' in choosing her partner while her partner unconsciously selects her to contain inadequate parts of himself experienced when comparing himself to aspects of this shared idealised internal father.

'Shared internal image' in this chapter refers primarily to the structure of the shared internal phantasy which informs the relationships between the mother, nanny and the baby. One such example of this would be when the nanny and mother's meticulously performed routine of child care is permeated by the image of the 'efficient caregiver numb to the baby's feelings'. This shared internal image may be a portrayal of a repressed, ongoing infantile experience of relating to a shared internal 'brick wall' mother who maintains no intimate contact with the infantile self. Consciously the mother and nanny may be working together in caring for baby in a very conscientious way. Naturally there can be changes in the evolving nature of the shared internal images, but generally there are visible trends in the shared internal dramas existing within mother–nanny and baby interactions.

This is an introduction to the way I develop a notion of shared internal images within the nanny–mother–baby interaction. In referring to the nanny I am often describing interactions which could as easily refer to au pairs, baby-sitters, grandmothers and other relatives, or mature siblings who are so frequently present in some cultures as the auxiliary caregivers. Also, in mentioning the mother or the parent I am often referring to a person whom I, in my culturally biased way, perceive to have the task of fulfilling the maternal functions of providing nurturing, physical comfort, security, receiving distressed aspects of the infantile self and, through thinking about the experience, modulating mental pain. I am also assuming that a father may often perform maternal functions while maintaining a distinct and separate role as father in relation to the baby.

I shall now describe six shared internal images frequently encountered in observing infants with nannies in their families, before going on to explore them in more detail in the remainder of the chapter.

Shared internal image: a nursing communion

The primary figure, usually the mother, is acknowledged as being particularly important and her relationship to the infant is felt to be irreplaceable. Some of mother's role of cherishing, nourishing, understanding and protecting the baby can also be undertaken by other caregivers, whilst they acknowledge the crucial importance of the infant's primary relationship to the mother. The shared image of 'a nursing communion' is one in which the caregiver gives meaning to the infant's feelings in relationships with caregivers who have different emotional significance to the baby. The infant thus develops the capacity to tolerate and forgive the caregiver for the occurrence of delays, absences and other frustrations.

Shared internal image: undifferentiated caregivers providing relief

The caregiver provides the infant with relief from distress and provides physical comfort. Acknowledgement of separation and feelings of loss in relation to a specific caregiver is absent, for there is no notion of an infant having a unique relationship with a particular attachment figure.

Shared internal image: placatory caregiver

The efficient caregiver is oblivious to the specific meaning of the infant's emotions. The infant's infantile pains are met in the most expedient way. In this way the infant is given the illusion that his needs are being considered, but in fact he is simply being placated. There is emotional distance in relation to any excruciating, intense emotional experiences, of both the caregiver and the infant.

Shared internal image: blessed or blamed caregiver

The caregiver should immediately gratify the infant's basic needs. If this gratification does not take place, the caregiver becomes a bad, cruel, caregiving figure who is felt to be guilty of neglect and is therefore blamed. The concept of developing a capacity to experience, tolerate and understand emotional discomfort does not exist. Idealisation and blaming are replacements for containment which is feared because it involves too much psychic pain.

Shared internal image: coupling cruel to the baby

Within the context of the family, there is a shared view that coupling between two figures is simply cruel to the 'left-out baby' figure. This 'left-out baby' figure could exist within any third person, baby, mother, nanny or father.

Shared internal image: the supportive couple

A couple is allowed to be together, meeting each other's basic emotional needs while 'holding in mind' the infantile needs of the third person, the 'baby-part' residing in the baby, or another family figure. In particular, the Oedipal parental couple is allowed to exist in a situation in which the united loving father and mother are allowed to provide erotic satisfaction to one another, and to cooperate in bringing up their children and in providing security to the infant. Even though the infant might simultaneously experience frustration at being left out, he is able to maintain an experience of his parents lovingly united and affectionately concerned about his well-being.

These shared internal images become apparent if one closely observes the ongoing pattern of the interaction between the family and the nanny. I use my emotional experiences in hearing an infant observation seminar student present and discuss the meetings with the baby and the family. While listening to the student observer, who is also part of the family interaction, my counter-transference responses to the presentation delineate shared internal images. These shared internal images, present in the mother–nanny–baby interaction, form the themes of a drama enacted on the stage of my mind.

Simultaneously I visualise some of the shared internal images created through the interactions between the students, me and the student observer. At times, undigested experiences from the shared internal images in the family are 'mirrored' in the interaction of the seminar.

For example, at the beginning of the first term, a student brought an observation in which the mother and a relatively new nanny agreed that mother would 'sneak out' in an attempt to prevent her two-month-old baby from noticing her departure. However, the minute mother disappeared, baby Mary began wailing. The nanny began jiggling a variety of noisy rattles in front of baby's face to distract her from being distressed by mother's departure. In response to this, baby stiffened her whole body, with her arms waving restlessly in front of her face and her legs kicking rapidly. The mother and nanny were attempting to evade some perceptions that the baby would get agitated and experience mother as an unkind and uncaring, absent figure. The nanny was distracting and placating baby Mary whose piercing cries revealed her experience of the world as a 'bad place'. Baby was virtually inconsolable when mother departed.

In this new observation seminar, with many anxieties of how the group would settle together with me, the new teacher, I experienced an immediate tendency on the part of the group to interact around this shared internal image of 'The Blessed or Blamed Caregiver'. This image involves the caretaker in being perceived as very good if absolutely meeting the baby's wishes or being perceived as a bad, cruel, unresponsive parental figure who is guilty of neglect if the baby experiences any frustration.

The seminar discussion veered towards criticising the nanny for being inadequate. The students were very critical of both mother and the nanny for 'being sneaky' about mother's departures. As I began to understand this tendency to criticise, I was able to talk about new experiences felt by the baby with the new observer present. There were new experiences for the nanny, likewise, with the observer watching her. I compared this with the immediate moment in the seminar in which we were all learning to work together at the beginning of a new term. Also, I attempted to enable the seminar members to identify with the anxieties present in the mother and nanny and to understand the nature of the difficulties which this pair, mother and nanny, had in understanding and experiencing the depth of baby's protest and distress about 'the bad, absent mother' created in baby's mind.

SHARED INTERNAL IMAGES: SOME EXAMPLES

Shared internal image: the nursing communion

Ideally, as I see it, the parents and the nanny whom they choose to look after their baby would have a certain shared internal image of the infant needing a primary caretaker who cherishes, nourishes, caresses and creates the opportunity for a nursing communion in which delays and shortcomings can be understood, tolerated and forgiven. The role of the nanny would be clearly defined to assist the mother in this task of containing intense emotions in the infant. The nanny would simultaneously be acknowledging to herself and to the baby the importance of the relation-ship to the parents, while at the same time the parents would be accepting of nanny's important emotional significance to the baby.

Here is an example from Mark, an infant who regularly screamed just before falling asleep at night. His mother had just hired a nanny the previous week. The previous day she had left Mark in the care of the nanny for six hours while she went to work for the first time.

Baby Mark: seven months
Mother and nanny are sitting together having breakfast. Held in mother's arms, baby attentively searches mother's face and then nanny's face. When nanny laughs, baby suddenly bursts into tears and, terrified, he screams. When mother holds him tightly with his head resting against her shoulder, baby sobs. Gradually baby's cries subside and he glances again at the eyes of nanny whereupon he recommences his screaming. This sequence is repeated four times.

Nanny perceives that through her laugh she has become a 'monster figure' for baby. Mother, feeling very guilty about her decision to leave baby in order to work, cannot bear to think about the emotional significance of Mark's cries. She describes how the baby is teething. However, she searches for some somatic meaning, saying: 'Mark may have a stomach ache. Maybe he needs his nappy changing.' The older, very experienced nanny begins to play peek-a-boo with baby.

Covering her face with a hanky nanny says, 'Gone away.' Then, uncovering her face she adds, 'Here she is.' She slowly repeats this game, while allowing baby time to tug away the hanky hiding her face. 'Mummy goes away. Mummy comes back. Go away. Come back. Hello. Goodbye. Hello', says nanny while alternately hiding and showing her face. Tentatively baby begins to smile when nanny's face reappears from behind the hanky.

Through this play mother realises that baby had some fears of separating from her and she acknowledges this in her discussion with the nanny. In this situation one sees how the nanny is able to recognise the importance of the separation from mother, for baby and mother. She is able to stay with and accept the baby's terror of a bad persecuting object projected into her laughing face and give meaning to the baby's internal experience. Baby Mark gradually feels able to work through some of his rage, and consequent anxieties about his good mother turning into a bad mother when mother changes the baby's routine and goes to work, thus leaving him for an unusually long time in the care of a relatively new nanny. Baby Mark's anger and fear of separation has provoked too much guilt in mother. This guilt prevented her from acknowledging his feelings. The nanny, however, was able to elaborate Mark's anxieties and mitigate some of the fierceness of his projections into the open 'monster mouth and eyes' of the nanny.

Mother has chosen a very empathic, competent nanny who assists the mother in the task of containing the intense feelings of the infant. When baby cries, both mother and nanny attempt to work together to give meaning to the baby's distress. The shared image of a nursing communion informed mother's choice of nanny and nanny's acknowledgement of the baby's primary attachment to mother. Through the play with baby, the nanny seemed to enable baby to restore his experience of a good mother.

The role definition of the nanny as being a very important figure assisting in the caregiving tasks implies that gratitude and admiration for her caregiving functions can arise. If the mother and nanny are able to meet the baby's emotional needs, the baby's attachment to them as significant, loved caregivers becomes more obvious. This increases the risk that unless they are able to remain located in their mature parental role and identify with baby, the nanny and mother may experience envy and jealousy in the infantile structures of their personality. These feelings may interfere with the shared task of nurturing, loving and understanding the baby. Dr John Bowlby (1970, personal communication) indicated that it was the unworked-through infantile emotions of envy and jealousy which often led mothers to choose short-stay nannies and inadequate nannies, while minimising the opportunities for more adequate caregiving for their babies. In particular, he stated how difficult it was for a mother who had sense of inadequacy to tolerate her own baby's attachment and love for a nanny with good capacities to mother the baby.

Shared internal image: undifferentiated caregivers providing relief

It is these infantile emotions of envy and jealousy which influence the formation of the shared internal image of 'Undifferentiated Caregivers Providing Relief'. This shared internal image is one in which the caregiver provides the infant with relief from distress, and provides physical comfort; absent, however, is any acknowledgement of an infant having a unique relationship with a specific attachment figure, which involves responses to separations and loss of that person. This internal image shared by mother and nanny includes the possibility of complete substitution of mother for nanny or nanny for mother, with no differentiation between the two in the baby's heart and mind. This shared internal image is present in the following observations of baby Barry.

Baby Barry was born into a professional family who already had a 5-year-old daughter. Mother did not work during the first two years of Barry's life, but she and a succession of three nannies shared his care during this time. There was no specific delineation of responsibilities of the caregivers so that when Barry cried, either mother or nanny would appear. Likewise, without any routine or any warning given to Barry, mother or nanny would disappear for several hours. Nevertheless, Barry maintained a very close relationship with his mother and the pair were obviously delighted in each other's company. This persisted throughout the two years of the observation.

Barry: four weeks
Mother holds baby to her with his head in the hollow of her neck. For a few minutes she rubs his back with slow gentle movements of her hand. Baby looks extremely content being held by mother. In this moment of intimacy mother, stroking baby's head tenderly says, 'This is all very time-consuming.' After a few minutes she lays baby in his cot, covering him over with a sheet. Baby begins to squirm, wave his arms in the air and make little bleating sounds. Mother stands for a moment with her hand resting on his chest and then departs.

Baby Barry lies quietly for a few seconds, then he 'stiffens' and screws up his face before crying with protest and fear. Soon the nanny arrives and stands beside the cot, looking down at Barry. He squirms a little more vigorously and his cries become louder. After a while the nanny picks him up and like mother had done previously, she holds his head in the hollow of her neck. Nanny then pats baby's bottom so hard that it makes the observer wince.

Baby continues to cry unremittingly after mother's absence. The nanny is disgruntled and somewhat persecuted by not knowing what Barry wants and needs. She says, 'What do you want Barry? Shall I change your nappy? You are a pain. Why don't you go to sleep. You are too noisy.' The nanny then feeds baby, changes his nappy, and makes him do peddling movements with his legs. In response Barry has hiccups which engulf his entire body.

Responding to Barry's underlying distress presents a problem for nanny. If she acknowledges that mother is extremely important to Barry, that he does not consider his nanny as being identical to mother, nor of equal importance to him, nanny has the problem of her own identity. She must feel worthwhile enough as a person to accept Barry's definition of the current situation – that nanny is not the one he wants or desires most. Feeling inadequate and insecure, nanny functions with these premises: 'Being with nanny is the same as being with mother. Mother is not needed. Now nanny is as good as mother.' In this way the nanny denies, rather than contains, Barry's genuine distress. Barry's hiccupping seems to be a sign of tension linked with nanny's activities performed in lieu of containing his unbearable pain of losing mother.

As is often the case, this mother found a nanny who had a similar personality structure to herself. Although mother is extremely tender with baby, she is often so overwhelmed with the intense attachment existing between them that she tends to deny baby's distress in separating from her. This denial frees mother to pursue her own plans. When baby is five months old, mother and father go on a week's holiday in the sun. Nanny and baby stay with maternal grandmother but the grandmother and the nanny don't see eye-to-eye.

When mother returns, the nanny is immediately replaced by a new nanny. Baby Barry is overjoyed to see mother when she returns from her holiday.

Barry: five months

Baby protests at being offered his bottle by the new nanny. When mother takes him and cuddles him, he takes the bottle readily and looks quite settled but when mother talks to nanny, he cries and wriggles about, protesting about losing mother's attention. When mother leaves baby to get the pram, he turns and gazes in mother's direction until she returns.

A few days after mother's return, baby is ill with a high temperature of 103°. His pale, translucent face is distorted by his sharp, complaining cries. The doctor diagnoses meningitis and baby is placed in hospital for eight days.

Barry: eleven months

Baby has a very differentiated response to mother and his third nanny. When the observer arrives, baby clings anxiously to the nanny. After a while when mother comes home he rapidly crawls towards her and grabs her legs. As soon as she bends down towards him, baby curls his arms around her neck and excitedly begins to bounce up and down.

Barry is a baby who has formed a strong, pleasurable attachment to his mother, He has delineated a 'good mother' who feeds him, keeps him clean, cuddles him and loves him. During times of separation from her, he is sometimes able to hold on to the internal image of a good mother. However, neither mother nor the nannies whom she chooses are able to remain responsive to Barry's helplessness, terror and rage, which beset him at the moment of mother's unpredictable absences. Also, no one has acknowledged the psychological importance to Barry of the permanent departures of the two previous nannies.

My impression is that shared denial of the importance of separation and loss of significant caregivers contributed to this baby's psychosomatic expression of emotional conflicts. We can note the pattern of Barry's responses to separation during his first two years. In the early weeks of life, baby protests against the change of caretaker, from mother to nanny, by crying inconsolably and vomiting. Nanny is not able to contain and acknowledge the source of his distress. At four and a half months, baby is

weaned. As babies often do, he protests against the bottle being introduced. Mother feels his anger about the 'lost breast' but does not register
at a deep emotional level, baby's sense of loss and rage about losing his
intimacy with her at the breast. The 'breast' filled with baby's rage turns
bad and is symbolised by 'the bad bottle'. Mother is unaware of baby's
resulting terror of 'the bad bottles' coming towards him. Barry develops
eczema. When Barry is five months old, mother goes for a one-week
holiday followed by the old nanny being replaced immediately; subsequently, baby gets meningitis. When the second nanny leaves, baby
immediately gets a series of colds. At thirteen months, Barry has persistent
sniffles and a wheezy chest. By two years he is diagnosed as having asthma.

My hypothesis is that Barry's illnesses are not simply coincidental with
the times of mother's absence and the nannies' departures. The baby's
uncontained feelings, in conjunction with mother's and each nanny's denial
of the importance of a particular relationship to mother and each different
nanny in his life, may contribute to the formation of his psychosomatic
illnesses. His body suffers what his psychic structure cannot bear. The
disappearance of two nannies in eleven months may also make a significant
contribution to baby's somatising of distress. Current child development
research (Main et al. 1985: 66–107) suggests that the infant internalises
unique types of attachment relationships with each caregiver. The infant
keeps the different relationships with the caregivers distinct in many ways.
For example, the infant may remain, according to Ainsworth's definitions
of attachments, securely attached to mother while insecurely attached to
father and/or the nanny.

N. Fox (1977) studied infants in the Israeli Kibbutzim. Both separation
and reunion with mother or *metapelet* (carer) created anxiety, for in most
children the *metapelet* was an attachment figure who was experienced as
being as important or more important than the mother. Losing the *metapelet* or losing mother caused a similar protest and consequent anxieties.
Reuniting with mother or the *metapelet*, while creating satisfaction and
joy, also involved losing 'a very significant other'. This may be a very
difficult fact for loving parents to digest when they come home from work,
keen to be with their baby. It may be very painful to remain in identification with the baby, acknowledging baby's attachment to the nanny, the
good experiences baby shared with the nanny while the parents were at
work, and baby's sense of loss in relation to the departure of the nanny
when the parents take over.

It is extremely hard for some biological mothers to acknowledge the
intense emotional significance the nanny has for their baby. This was
researched and discussed by Dr H.T. Hardin (1985). During a five-year
period, 31 out of 102 new patients he examined, and five patients in
psychoanalytic treatment, had distinct and significant primary surrogate
mother care in their infancies. Clinical examples limited to patients losing

nannies some time after their eighteenth month revealed that termination of surrogate caregiving was always experienced as traumatic. The image of the nanny was concealed by images of the biological mother, but in the course of therapy, the nanny emerged as having been distinct and significant in the patient's infancy. One factor which prolonged rather than ameliorated the child's trauma of separation from the nanny was the incapacity of the mother to acknowledge the profound emotional tie existing between her infant and the nanny. Also, the mother's denial of the disturbing circumstances surrounding the permanent termination of the contact between nanny and infant profoundly disturbed the psychological development of the infant.

More serious consequences of the denied impact of separation of nanny from the child occurred if the attachment to the nanny occurred before eighteen months and the separation occurred before three years. Primary psychological consequences of attachment and a loss of a surrogate, or an estrangement from the biological mother, contributed to an over-sensitivity to separation and loss in general. Hardin suggested that all these factors contributed to subsequent difficulties in forming intimate relationships.

Separation from an emotionally significant figure such as the nanny is problematic for the child. In view of this widely known fact, why is it that many mothers have so much difficulty in fully acknowledging the importance of the nanny as a person and as a significant caregiver for her child? My impression is that the importance of the nanny for the child is negated or denied in an attempt to evade unbearable painful feelings, such as guilt, that the nanny is providing care for the baby which the mother feels she would like to, or should provide. For example, when her fretful baby was left at home with the nanny and fell asleep peacefully, one mother became worried about whether or not her baby really loved her. Another mother said that when her baby was born, initially she was too upset to do the quiet things you do with a baby – walking her and talking with her. After she saw the nanny doing those peaceful activities, mother cried, saying: 'I couldn't do it because I was too depressed' (Hardin 1985: 624). Also, if the mother devalues the significance of the nanny she may not feel so envious of the nanny's important mothering capacities such as warmth, understanding and tolerance.

Shared internal image: the placatory caregiver

Perhaps more difficult to experience as an observer is the shared internal image of an efficient caregiver who is oblivious to the specific meaning of the infant's emotions. The expedient caregiver meets the infant's emotional and physical needs with minimal emotional contact with the excruciating, intense emotional experiences of pleasure, joy, love, anger and sadness existing in either the caregiver or the infant.

For example, one young nanny described her life in a family saying she spends each day with two girls, blond-haired Bernadette, 2 years, and red-haired Rebecca, who is eight months old. The nanny and the children have a nursery which has a separate access to the garden and laundry. They do not go to the rest of the house unless invited. The nanny has the exclusive role of taking care of the children, preparing their meals, doing their laundry and ironing and cleaning the nursery. Mother has a busy social life and meets the children one hour each day for 'playtime'. The children are with their parents one and a half days at the weekend when the nanny has time off. Generally, the nanny and children can be found in the nursery wing which is upstairs in a separate part of the family mansion.

> Nanny and mother make time each morning to discuss the children. One morning they discuss the previous night in which 2-year-old Bernadette had awakened three times. They can't discover any reason for her crying and come to the conclusion, 'Who knows, it's just one of those things that she continues to do.' As soon as the nanny returns to the nursery she hears an exuberant voice call out – 'Nanny, Bernie awake. Nanny! Nanny!' Bernadette is grinning from ear to ear and bouncing with delight to see the nanny who cuddles her and kisses her.
>
> At night the younger sister, eight-month-old Rebecca, cries after she is put to bed. Nanny says there is no apparent cause for the crying and Rebecca generally is comforted with a hug, cuddle and kiss. Some days Nanny feels Bernadette, the 2-year-old, is a 'real pain' and 'drives her up the wall', whining and crying and deliberately annoying her with behaviour 'she knows is naughty'. Rebecca cries after a walk outside in the park, not wanting to come back into the house on a day when the mother is away for most of the day shopping.

What is conveyed in this observation is how the parents and the nanny have agreed on a role definition for the nanny which denies the significance of the primary figure, the mother. Meanwhile the parents involve themselves in other activities. The nanny says rather poignantly, 'Sometimes I feel trapped, I feel like a single mother. I wish I had more time to myself.'

The definition of the nanny as the substitute mother has been agreed upon by the parents and the nanny. Both the parents and the nanny seem to lack any notion that the children may have consciously accepted the role of the nanny, allowing their parents freedom to be separate from them most of the time. Yet the girls still feel some vague yearning for something indefinable which is lacking – the mother, the father – in their day-to-day lives. When the ritual of nanny replacing mother has been accepted by all the caregivers, it seems difficult for this nanny to consider the meaning of the children's tears. Unsupported, she cannot bear their missing her, nor can she get in touch with their yearning or fears linked with the absence of their parents during the week. Instead, the nanny associates 2-year-old Bernadette's whining and crying with 'being a brat' and 'being naughty'. Likewise, she cannot comprehend eight-month-old Rebecca's crying as she lies in bed, for the nanny does not view her own presence or mother's as important to Rebecca. It is too painful for nanny to perceive that the mother's absence is very important to the children. Denial of the importance of mothering and significant attachments to parents and nanny is a shared defence on the part of both the nanny and the parents. The nanny comments: 'I like this job a great deal. The mother and I get along very well.'

In listening to these comments of the nanny, I wondered about the routine of caregiving to the children which involved so little of mother's time. Looming into view was the large mansion, in which the nanny was immediately placed in care of newly born Rebecca, out of hearing distance from her parents. I imagined how it was for mother to greet baby who knew so little of her while she knew so little of the new baby. I recalled Ilse Westheimer's (1970: 9) comments on how the mother may experience herself as unimportant to the baby if the baby is not immediately responsive to her. The mother can feel a no-good mother and her communication with the baby can lessen while the nanny is relied upon more heavily.

Ilse Westheimer (1970: 3–10) has shown how the response of a mother to a child during periods of separation can easily parallel the child's responses to separation. The infant becomes detached from the mother and more involved with a substitute caregiver. As this occurs the mother is prone to become detached from the infant, losing some of her former maternal responsiveness. A mother may experience a sense of loss in separating from her child, but then find that her child is remote and apathetic when she returns home. This can be a source of intense guilt and incredible pain; the mother may retreat to a more remote, detached relationship to the child. In these situations, a sensitive nanny can support the mother who cannot bear the guilt over loss of a good relationship with the child and pain about the loss of intimacy between mother and child. However, this would involve the nanny in retaining a deep belief in the importance of the mother for the infant and understanding the baby and mother's experience surrounding separations. Instead of being 'the placatory caregiver', oblivious to the specific meaning of the children's distress and mother's pain, the nanny would be identifying with the mother's pain which was prompting mother's denial and defensive withdrawal from her infant.

Shared internal image: coupling cruel to the baby

While in the previous situation, intense and overwhelming feelings were defended against through 'emotional distancing' and placating gestures, in other parent–nanny interactions there emerges a very strong infantile jealousy. Here the shared internal image is that coupling, with exclusion of a third figure, is cruel to the 'left-out baby'. The feeling of being the 'left-out baby' can be experienced by baby, another family figure or the nanny.

Here is a vignette of Jack and his nanny which illustrates this shared internal image:

Baby Jack

Jack is the newly born third child of a suburban American family. His mother is a housewife actively involved in a social life with her husband who is a businessman. The nanny does everything for Jack except feed him. She bathes him, changes him and sleeps in the nursery with him. This means that mother's routine of cooking, shopping and socialising is barely disturbed by baby's birth. Mother is not aware of Jack's crying during the night and remaining awake in nanny's arms for long periods.

Mother shares nanny's view that nanny is the expert and should be in charge, although nanny is younger than mother and actually less experienced with children. Nanny has decided to use a watch to time the baby's feeding at each breast. Nanny is also relied upon by mother to remember on which breast mother should start the feeding. In having such control over mother and baby, nanny interferes with mother and baby's more spontaneous rhythm of being together.

During Jack's feeds, nanny tends to talk to mother. This creates a disturbance to Jack and maintains a distance between him and his mother. Sometimes, in a distressingly intrusive way, nanny cuts Jack's fingernails while he is feeding. It appears that she cannot bear the closeness of the feeding couple and her exclusion from it.

On the other hand, nanny enjoys her own intimate moments with Jack and there is a possibility that nanny's cuddling of Jack during the night positively reinforces his wakefulness. There is a hint that both nanny and baby are unable to tolerate the absence of the intimacy which is shared by the parental couple, and their night-time cuddling is a placation of their frustration of not being part of a couple. Nanny insists that Jack is at his best alone with her in the morning. It seems that nanny unconsciously experiences jealousy not only of the adult couple, but also of the couple, mother and baby. Her jealousy of mother and competition with her not only prevents the nanny from allowing mother some privacy with baby but also from assisting mother to acknowledge both her own mothering capacities or her importance to the baby.

Here are two scenes typical of the first few weeks of baby's life, which illustrate nanny's interference with mother's mothering:

> *Baby Jack: two weeks old*
> Jack is feeding at the breast, he is looking slightly above the breast, watching the space where mother's face can be seen when she turns to look at him. When mother is not looking directly at him, he gazes vacantly into the space. Shortly, mother is engaged in a conversation. Jack continues to suck in a relaxed way, but as mother's attention continues to be directed to the nanny, he gradually becomes more self-absorbed and tired.

At times it may be natural for baby to get drowsy during a feed, but often drowsiness at these moments seems to be a protection against stress or lack of attentiveness from mother.

By way of contrast to this observation where Jack stares into the empty space and then gets drowsy when mother is absorbed with the nanny, here is an observation typical of times when mother manages to be alone with Jack.

> *Baby Jack: three weeks*
> Mother and baby spent a lot of time gazing at each other with real concentration. Mother occasionally speaks to baby as she feeds him. Baby remains active in his sucking and alert after the feed. He looks in an active searching way into mother's eyes.

There seems to be another problem in this mother–nanny relationship. Mother is unable to acknowledge or at times use her own capacities as a mother. She frequently emphasises her own incompetence in her discussions with the observer. She refers to herself as 'a fumbling mom', although she is very in touch with baby's emotions when she is with him and capable in her handling of him. It is a common experience for some mothers, who are perhaps envious of their nanny's mothering capacities, to subsequently feel they 'have nothing to offer' their babies, for envy creates this experience of 'having nothing inside'. Simultaneously the nanny maintains her position of being 'the expert mother' who shows this mother of three children how to do things, and tells her what to do in a way that continually interferes with the 'mother–baby couple'.

In these observations, we see several problems which intrude upon potentially good caregivers of Jack. First, nanny identifies with a 'super-mom' (Dartington and Magagna 1994: 144) who can do everything perfectly while projecting into mother all her uncertainty and lack of understanding of baby's needs. This kind of projective identification is a defence used when nanny cannot contain the stress of managing all the parts of her own personality. She needs to feel very confident in order to maintain her identity as 'the good nanny'. Also, nanny's own unresolved infantile conflicts prompt her to be jealous of baby's relationship with mother. She wants either mother for herself or Jack for herself for she cannot bear being the excluded 'third figure'.

Shared internal image: the supportive couple

With this shared internal image, the caregiver is quite different. Here there is a shared image that a couple – mother and father as well as baby and another caregiver – are allowed to be together. Baby's deep emotional needs by necessity are being met for some time by the nanny. The third person, the mother, is needing to find ways of having her own emotional needs met before she can reinstate herself as part of a close mother–child couple. I have only implicitly shown the nanny's capacity to acknowledge and accept mother's need for re-entering her adult world with her husband and colleagues, but this was also present in the observation which follows of Sacha, a beautiful baby, the first child born to her mother, an Italian opera singer, and her father, an international management consultant.

Baby Sacha: two weeks
Baby sucks rhythmically at mother's breast while mother gently strokes her cheek. Mother watches her baby with rapture, as though transfixed by the pleasant experience of the baby at the breast. Mother remains still, allowing baby to suck and then rest with her mouth holding the nipple. Later she tenderly rocks Sacha in her lap. Following the feed, mother expresses her delight that baby is sucking powerfully and eagerly on the breast.

By one month, baby never comes off the breast voluntarily. She finds everything distressing unless she is at mother's breast or with a person. Mother and baby behave in a 'harmonious and practised way' together. There she can find solace. Sacha's eyes wander in an unfocused way towards mother's face as mother is talking. Mother and observer discuss how Sacha isn't following people or moving objects with her eyes in the way babies of her age should. Mother decides to have Sacha's eyes checked by a paediatrician. Meanwhile, in quite a relentless way, she begins to elicit Sacha's attention by moving toys in front of her face. Because mother intuitively feels Sacha is handicapped in some way, she is trying to give her a big dose of stimulation as recommended by some of the books for handicapped babies.

Aware of being extremely anxious about the normality of her baby, mother cannot concentrate on her music and for this reason she cancels her future singing engagements. Nevertheless, mother and baby lose a satisfying rapport with one another. Mother says, 'It's difficult to keep in touch. Without the baby's look I don't know what I'm getting back from her.'

When baby is four months, she is diagnosed as having a very uncommon congenital illness, which includes blindness as well as the possibility of mental retardation and other life-threatening physical problems. Naturally, mother is extremely sad because she does not have a 'normal baby'. She cannot bear the pain of facing her not-seeing daughter. Also, she feels disheartened about the baby's slow motor development. In this state, mother is able to respond only briefly to baby's crying. She finds herself unable to be close to baby and embrace her for long when she screams or cries intensely.

Baby Sacha: four months
Sacha screams loudly and collapses face downwards onto the rug. Mother says, 'Oh, dear, and I had so wanted to show off your new trick.' She picks up screaming baby and holds her briefly before placing her in a sitting up position on her beanbag.

Around this time Mother arranged for a nanny to take over some of the care of baby. Initially, the presence of the nanny enables mother to flee from the baby and get re-involved in her professional career. Not surprisingly, mother finds that because singing requires her to be very emotionally involved in the music, she must protect herself by embarking on music research. The nanny's arrival means that mother is free to become even more distant and out of touch with baby Sacha. But the nanny is attached to both mother and baby. Although she has a great sense of pride in caring for Sacha and forming a loving relationship with her, the nanny is also keen to give mother opportunities to reconnect with her daughter, through sharing with mother some of her perceptions of the baby's love and attachment to mother.

Baby Sacha: ten months
When baby protests about being taken out of the bath, nanny knows what baby hates and fears. She talks to baby comfortingly while rubbing gently with a towel. Quite quickly, Sacha's plaintive wails diminish. Nanny kisses baby tenderly on her cheek and neck, saying, 'What a lovely little girl you are.' She says to the observer, 'I can't believe how attached you can become to a baby. I've looked after other children, but I've never felt like this about a child.' Baby then sucks loudly on a bottle nanny provides. After a while she begins crying. As the nanny picks her up and cuddles her, Sacha pushes her face into nanny's neck, placing her little hands against nanny's shoulders. Nanny says, 'Baby is much more cuddly now, she doesn't arch her neck and pull away as she used to with her mother and me.' Baby's cries gradually subside.

Over time nanny is able to establish a close tie with baby because she is not too disappointed or persecuted by baby's visual non-responsiveness and her difficulty in being comforted. She does not feel rejected by baby's pulling away from her as she tries to hold and comfort her. This is very different from mother's sense of persecution and rejection of baby.

As the consequence of being physically held and emotionally contained by the nanny, baby is able to develop an internal image of a trustworthy, strong comforting 'mother figure' who can bear her anger and distress. The picture of a 'good internal mother' – derived to a considerable extent from experiences with the nanny – enables baby to adapt to her mother's demands for her to perform. During the next six to eight months baby and mother are gradually able to re-establish an old connection that has been broken through the trauma of baby's partial blindness.

Baby Sacha: eighteen months
When Sacha is eighteen months old, one year after nanny's arrival, the situation is dramatically changed. Mother says she is 'enjoying Sacha now'. Mother has regained her confidence and cheerfulness. Now baby is self-possessed and responsive to mother.

Mother begins a nursery rhyme, 'Ring-a-ring-a-roses', Sacha adds 'tissue, tissue, all fall down'. Mother responds with squeals of delight and cuddles which thrill baby.

The nanny has helped mother through the crisis of being unable to be intensely involved with her partially blind baby. This supportive link between mother and baby has been recreated. Also mother finds she can resume her music recitals, for again she is in touch with her emotions, a necessary experience for her success as a singer and as a mother.

These observations illustrate how, unlike mother, nanny can bear baby's terror, unresponsiveness and handicap. This good relationship with nanny is subsequently transferred to baby's relationship to mother. Because nanny loves baby and identifies with baby's needs, including baby's need for mother, the nanny does not compete with mother. We see here how a loving couple – mother and baby, are encouraged to form a more intimate relationship through the nanny's support.

ASSESSMENT: REMEMBERING THE NANNY

I have shown the significant influence of shared internal images in the nanny–mother–baby relationship in the infant's developing personality. One of my reasons for doing this is to encourage therapists doing an assessment of a child to patiently persist in developing a full, detailed picture of the child's unconscious and external relationships with each of the caregivers in his life, including the past and present nannies. Often the parents have not consciously accepted the depth of the attachment between the nanny and their child because they are evading their jealousy of the nanny, and the child's pain of separation, which may have occurred in relation to the nannies in his life. The child's pattern of bearing mental pain and relating to significant people in his life may be linked with his experience of being 'mothered' by both mother and several nannies. For this reason, it is important to remember the nanny when making an assessment of the child's emotional development and personality structure.

Here is a vignette illustrating some of the difficulties and benefits of taking the nanny's role into consideration when meeting with the child's parents during an assessment. This is description provided by Mrs Martha Harris who headed the Child Psychotherapy Training at the Tavistock Clinic.

Mrs Harris (1984: 32) illustrated the importance of moving beyond generalised statements about the child and nanny's relationship to very detailed observations of the 'baby-in-the-present' linked to 'the-baby-in-the-past'. She discussed a consultation with a family who were worried about their fourteen-month-old child John. John was a delicate-featured white-faced little boy with his father's large forehead and intelligent eyes and with the sensitive expressions and distant composure of the mother. He was keeping his young parents awake all night with head-banging and constant demands for attention. At ten months John, who previously had slept and eaten well, began to awaken two or three times in the night, refusing to return to his bed.

Mother said that she had had two changes of au pair, one when John was eight months old and the next when he was eleven months. John had been very attached to both girls, but mother did not think that his head-banging and sleeplessness could be connected with their disappearance as he was not very attached to his new au pair. Mrs Harris continued to explore John's early development until she could see the 'child from the past' in the present consultation. When she asked the mother to describe how John was with the au pairs, mother mentioned how attached John was to each of them. Mother added that he had not responded to either separation by expressing obvious distress. He did however begin head-banging and became sleepless around the time the departing second au pair was in a hysterical state about an unhappy love affair. What was important in this assessment was how Mrs Harris persisted in gathering details regarding the au pair's state of mind and John's responses to her. She did not simply rely on their mother's lack of acknowledgement of the au pairs' influence upon John's state of mind.

Gradually in the assessment, Mrs Harris noticed that when mother was in a distracted, distant relationship with John, he pulled a wastepaper basket violently towards himself, banged his upper lip hard, took a deep breath, closed his lips firmly and for a few seconds rubbed his forehead in a distressed, anxious way. She suggested that this seemed rather like

John's reaction to the pain of parting from the au pairs of whom he was so fond. At these times he had kept a stiff upper lip and held the painful feeling to himself. However, at night he had a violent outlet through crying and head-banging, suggesting that he had a nasty emotional experience in his head.

Mrs Harris had succeeded in enabling the mother to see more fully her 'child-in-the-present' through noting details of his 'stiff upper lip' and breath-holding as features of the 'child-in-the-past-still-present'. Also, she gave mother the opportunity to observe with more clarity and detail her 'child-in-the-past' in relation to the au pairs, their states of mind and departures. It was only through patiently creating a detailed observation together with the mother, that Mrs Harris was able to assist the parents in finding ways of deeply understanding their child's relationships to the pain of the departures and troubled states of mind of the au pairs.

CONCLUSION: THE IMAGE OF THE 'OTHER CAREGIVER' AS A SPACE FOR PROJECTIONS FROM THE INNER WORLD

The parents hold within themselves a certain image of an internal mother, a caregiver for the infantile parts of themselves. This influences their conscious choice of a nanny who will best portray their image of 'a good caregiver'. The selected nanny brings her own 'internal caregiver', her own internal mother with whom she identifies in mothering the baby. It is the relationship between the nanny and the parents which brings into play different 'shared internal images' of caregiving for the infant. Diane Wulfsohn (1988) in 'The impact of the South African nanny on a young child' shows how the parents and nannies have the opportunity to become supportive to each other or rivalrous about the attachment and care of the children. As the mother and nanny's relationship increases in warmth and closeness, there is trend towards the nanny having a more facilitating, positive caregiving relationship to the baby. A good, supportive relationship between the mother and a nanny facilitates their identification with loving, sensitive internal parental images, who can experience the infant's emotions, hold them in mind and give proper emotional significance to the baby's attachment and dependence on the state of mind of other caregivers.

What becomes obvious in observing infants is that the baby's intense emotional experience of joy and pleasure with a caregiver or the baby's piercing pain about not being understood can elicit the caregiver's own unworked-through infantile relationship to parental figures. When the baby experiences joy with a nanny or mother, the other caregiver can feel useless or jealous, rather than pleased in identification with the baby. When the baby is in a crisis, the caregiver can easily identify with the baby's anger, hatred, life-threatening anxieties and blame the 'other one', either the nanny or the mother for not being 'an adequate mother-figure'. This can lead to paranoid anxieties with each caregiver fearing the unvoiced criticisms of the other. Through these experiences is born the unconscious rivalry with the mothering capacities in the nanny or mother. This unconscious rivalry can interfere with giving full emotional significance to the level of attachment which the baby experiences when a significant caregiver, a parent or nanny, is arriving, departing or providing care for the baby. Acute anxiety states in baby at night can suggest that the baby's daytime experiences are not being sufficiently contained and elaborated upon in the daytime by the significant caregivers.

Raising a family requires the parents to spend time discussing and understanding their child and their relationship with him. Likewise, the joint caregiving between the partners, parents and nanny, requires continual, detailed observation, discussion and consideration of their roles in relationship to the infant. In this chapter I suggest that the most helpful role of nanny is to promote the development of intimacy and continuity of a vital like between the parents and the baby. At the same time I suggest that it is essential for the parents to acknowledge the important role of the nanny as a significant attachment figure for the infant. Also, I have implied that parents and therapists need to understand the baby's primitive emotional attachment to and dependency upon the different qualities of each of his significant caregivers. This involves noticing and accepting baby's grief and intense attachments throughout his life, and holding in mind the crucial fact that a different caregiver, either parent or nanny, cannot completely replace a baby's unique relationship with another significant caregiver. Finally, this chapter is intended to highlight the need to comprehend the significant influence of the nanny–parent 'shared internal images' on the developing personality of the infant.

ACKNOWLEDGEMENTS

I would like to thank Dr Irene Fairbairn and Mrs Heather Pritchard for their observations which are in this paper.

REFERENCES

Bowlby, J. (1970) Personal communication with his Child Development Seminar Group in the Tavistock Clinic, London.

Dartington, A. and Magagna, J. (1994) 'Making a space for parents', in S. Box *et al.* (eds) *Crises in Adolescence*, New York: Jason Aronson.

Deutsch, H. (1963) 'A two-year-old boy's first love comes to grief', in *Neuroses and Character Types*, New York: International University Press (first published 1919).

Dicks, H. (1967) *Marital Tensions*, London: Routledge and Kegan Paul.

Fenichel, O. (1954) 'The pregenital antecedents of the Oedipal complex', in *The Collected Papers of O. H. O. Fenichel*, first series, London: Routledge and Kegan Paul (first published 1930).

Fox, N. (1977) 'Attachment of kibbutz infants to mother and metapelet', *Child Development*, 48: 1228–1239.

Freud, A. (1946) *The Psychoanalytic Treatment of Children*, New York: International University Press.

Freud, S. (1954) *The Origins of Psychoanalysis: Letters to Wilhelm Fliess, Drafts and Notes: 1877–1902*, New York: Basic Books.

Hardin, H. T. (1985) 'On the vicissitudes of early primary surrogate mothering', *Journal of American Psychoanalytic Association*, 33: 609–629.

Hardin, H. T. (1986) 'On the vicissitudes of Freud's early mothering and alienation from his biological mother', paper presented at 40th anniversary of the Menninger School of Psychiatry, Topeka, Kansas. Also found in a revised version in *Psychoanalytic Quarterly*, 1988, 57: 72–86.

Harris, M. (1984) *Thinking about Infants and Young Children*, Strath Tay, Perthshire: Clunie Press.

Main, M., Kaplan, N. and Cassidy, J. (1985) 'Security in infancy, childhood, and adulthood: a move to the level of representation', in *Growing Points of Attachment Theory and Research*, edited by Inge Bretherton and Everett Waters, Monographs of the Society for Research in Child Development No. 209, 50, 1–2: 66–107.

Meltzer, D. (1994) *Sincerity and Other Works*, edited by Alberto Hahn, London: Karnac Books.

Sachs, J. J. (1971) 'The maid: her importance in child development', *Psychoanalytic Quarterly*, 40: 469–484.

Weisner, T. S. and Gallimore, R. (1977) 'My brother's keeper: child and sibling caretaking', *Journal of Current Anthropology*, 18: 2, 169–190.

Westheimer, Ilse (1970) 'Changes in response of mother to child during periods of separation', *Social Work*, 27: 3–10.

Winnicott, D. W. (1976) 'Ego distortion in terms of true and false self', in *The Maturational Processes and the Facilitating Environment*, New York: International University Press (first published 1960).

Wulfsohn, D. (1988) 'The impact of the South African nanny on the young child', unpublished dissertation, London: Tavistock Clinic Library.

Chapter 4

The meaning of difference
Race, culture and context in infant observation

Lynda Ellis

This chapter explores the particular contribution which infant observation can make to an understanding of how meaning is attributed to difference, how it might be experienced and its impact in terms of internal and external realities.

Uniquely perhaps, the observational method allows one to examine at close quarters the ways in which specific cultural codes impact on a particular individual in a family context. It is precisely because observing an infant is such an intimate encounter that the painstaking attention to detail can show how significant aspects of human interactions can be misunderstood, distorted or lost. The subsequent careful reflection on the attribution of meaning which takes place in seminar discussion of observation material is vital and informative in terms of examining the nature of difference.

One of the features of the observational experience is that it brings us into close contact not only with the common elements of human growth and development but also with the rich and infinitely variable differences which make up each individual human being. We can recognise, however, that within particular contexts, difference can be experienced as desirable or undesirable, and what in one arena attracts admiration can in another be a repository for feelings of exclusion, hate and fear. This of course extends beyond the individual to groups, communities and nation states.

Folklore and fairy tales can speak vividly to human experience and Hans Christian Andersen's classic tale of the silver shilling offers one way of looking at the world through different eyes. It is a tale where a newly minted coin finds itself in foreign parts and sets forth with optimism and excitement 'to get to know strange people and foreign customs'. What he meets is rejection and attributions of worthlessness which makes him lose sight of his intrinsic value and leads him to conclude that 'in the eyes of the world one has only the value the world chooses to put upon one'.

In my observation of a black baby born in Britain I had the experience of being the foreigner, the 'shilling' as it were in the world of this family's home as they were foreigners in my white world beyond their doors. This brought into sharp relief our respective socio-cultural codes, customs and expectations not only in terms of disparities but also in regard to common ground. Further, it highlighted the way in which a preoccupation with the cultural context of human experience can lead one to behave as if individuals have no internal world, denying the inner cultural milieu which is perpetually interacting with external realities.

Observations take place in a diverse socio-cultural and political context and one would expect there to be some reflection of this in the mix of those embarking on observational experience, either as observer or observed. In extending observation as a research and training method, it is important to recognise, in my view, that this necessarily involves some thinking and discussion about how the observation of a child of a particular racial and cultural history impacts on all those party to the process and how aspects of difference come to be thought about and interpreted.

Crucially, there is an additional dimension to conducting an infant observation in terms of the ways in which socio-cultural frameworks shape and give meaning to our interpretations. The notion of childhood, for instance, as a distinct and discrete developmental period requiring special kinds of care and attention, education, entertainment and so on is so integral to a Western reality that one has to be reminded of just how contemporary a way of thinking this is. Such practices as baby farming, binding infants and dosing them with laudanum, viewing children as beings to be tolerated and controlled rather than cherished, even idolised, belong not to ancient but to recent history.

In the more complicated and sophisticated realm of judgements about what is good or bad, right or wrong for children, the potential for prejudice, value conflict and moralising is obvious. Debates about, for example, discipline, paternal and maternal responsibilities, single parenthood, sexual conduct, marriage (arranged or otherwise) and divorce are frequently characterised by a heatedness and polarisation which suggests they are rooted in part in deep-seated, irrational ideas, however well-informed the range of views expressed might appear to be. Ultimately, the observational method enables one not only to see what is before one's eyes but also to attend systematically to its meaning in a way which takes account of internal as well as external knowledge.

The observation material to be presented highlights the disturbing impact of an approach to mothering which has developed in one particular cultural context and is at odds with the expectations and infrastructure of a different socio-cultural environment. Observational sequences which proved difficult to process and/or which stirred especially strong feelings about racism and conflicting cultural codes will be explored with a particular focus on the interplay between internal and external factors. It will be evident that the family and thus, inevitably, I as observer, were exposed to a range of harsh and adverse circumstances, one dimension of this being a social and cultural isolation, especially in the early months of the baby's life.

This contextual component of cultural isolation will be seen to have its counterpart in relation to an internal sense of apartness and unconnected-ness as problems and issues to do with mother's capacity for reverie (Bion 1988: 36) and containment of her baby began to emerge. The concept of containment is explored elsewhere in this book but there are aspects which have particular relevance for this observation, notably the impact on mother and child of a lack of containment and its potential consequences in terms of personality development. Crucially, containment has an environ-mental context beyond that of the mother's state of mind and this in turn influences what she is able to make of the internal capacities she brings to mothering her baby.

The most difficult situation, and that which is most toxic in relation to mental life is where the mother, lacking adequate containment of herself, pushes back into the baby her own intolerable distress, producing a state described by Bion (1984: 116) as one of 'nameless dread'. Acknowledging the view that it is the mother's internal capacities for containment which are of primary significance – that is to say, the combination of constitutional factors, internal object relations and actual experiences of being parented – nonetheless certain external realities may have a profound impact on internal states. For example, the persecutory quality of experiences of racism which range from unspoken attributions of inferiority through to exclusion, rejection and racial attacks on individuals and communities may serve to amplify inner persecutory anxieties in a black mother and thus make it difficult, even impossible, for her to bear those which her baby might be trying to communicate.

Bick (1987: 116) brings another perspective to this concept of contain-ment, emphasising how the containing object is experienced concretely as a skin; this experience links with the infant's sensory relation to, and with, his mother. Harris (1987: 142) describes Bick's view of:

> the infant's need in his primary unintegrated state for an object that can hold the parts of the personality together, optimally the nipple in the mouth and the increasingly familiar holding, talking, smelling mother who meets his various sensual needs.

Of particular relevance to this observation material is Bick's consideration of what happens when what she terms this 'primal skin function' is imp-aired in some way, that is, when the infant's need for an object (the nipple-mother) that can hold the parts of the personality together is not met. She suggests that 'second skin' formation occurs 'when reliance and trust in an internal sustaining object is replaced by brittle independence of a muscular kind' (Harris 1987: 143). This creation of a sensory substitute for the skin container is problematic in terms of personality development since 'it may lead to a two-dimensional type of personality in which identification is of an adhesive kind, when mimicry and imitation of the surface qualities of people take the place of learning from experience' (Harris 1987: 143). There were striking examples in this observation of what appeared to be infantile and adult manifestations of such mechanisms the exploration of which proved surprisingly complex and troublesome, especially in relation to the significance of cultural factors.

To turn now to the observation, a brief introduction to the infant and his parents will be followed by material in four parts: 'Early days', 'Growing up', 'Moving on' and 'Coming through'. Baby Jaruba was born in 1990. His parents, Mr and Mrs Ekoku, are both of West African origin though of different tribal background and first language. (The term West African is used in an attempt to avoid identifying features appearing in the observation material in accordance with a commitment to confidentiality. It does not imply homogeneity in relation to African socio-cultural history and experience.) Before their arrival in Britain, the couple lived for some time in Germany where they had a well-established routine and circle of friends. Mrs Ekoku was immersed in her professional occupation and an active social life. Mr Ekoku was also a respected and well-paid professional and the move to England was originally explained to me as being con-nected with his work.

It became apparent, however that Mrs Ekoku's insecurities around the marital relationship and her pregnancy, coupled with growing fears about the rise of extreme right-wing politics and racism in Germany had been far more influential factors. Mr Ekoku had in fact taken a less than satisfactory job which was to have quite serious financial and morale implications and many months passed with little improvement in their circumstances. The family home initially was a rather gloomy, privately rented, terraced property in an area of the city with a sizeable ethnic minority population. They subsequently moved to a medium-rise council flat in an area of considerable social deprivation and barely concealed antagonism towards black families.

Mr and Mrs Ekoku did establish a number of social contacts, largely it seemed with white, middle-class professionals through their respective employment networks and they made efforts to sustain relationships made in Germany. However, their overwhelming experience of life in Britain, especially in the first months, seemed to be that of isolation and marginal-isation.

EARLY DAYS

My first meeting with Mrs Ekoku came a week or so before her expected date of delivery and there was some evidence that she was experiencing difficulty with her changed, that is, heavily pregnant, state. She was attempting to find work, attending interviews and so on, although almost at term, and her seemingly manic busy-ness led her to neglect herself in terms of adequate food and rest to the extent that, at one point, she collapsed in the city centre. This kind of detachment about what was happening in her body had, it seemed, a parallel in terms of how possible it was to keep her unborn baby in mind, and I was struck by the way in which potential difficulties about arranging a further meeting were, for her, connected with clashes with interview dates rather than the more or less imminent arrival of her baby.

Thinking about her attitude towards her pregnancy gave rise to the first of many periods of personal reflection and discussions with seminar colleagues about the cultural assumptions which I, as observer, might be making about appropriate behaviour and whether within another cultural context Mrs Ekoku's actions, that is, the priority given to financial security in relation to the baby's well-being, would be deemed entirely ordinary. Acknowledging this, however, we were still left with questions about her day-to-day experiences of a first pregnancy, her individual hopes and anxieties, her apparent tendency to agitation and flight, and the impact of all of this on the baby inside her. The following extract gives something of a flavour of this first meeting.

> Much of what Mrs Ekoku says about her pregnancy seems to be connected with arrangements and contacts, e.g., the National Childbirth Trust, and I have the growing sense that the baby is somehow incidental to whatever else is going on in her life. Her mind seems full of things she is doing or plans to do. I wonder if this is an ordinary process of familiarisation with a new city but there actually seems to be an impulsive purposelessness about her actions. At one point, as I am feeling a kind of breathlessness in myself, she says something to the effect of not having time to think and I have the sense of her baby not so much as a growing being in her mind rather as a series of tasks to be done, an overlay of a drive to accomplishment on the whole experience.

My next meeting with Mrs Ekoku was around eleven days after the birth and she told me movingly and in some detail how Jaruba was delivered by caesarean section after a protracted and distressing labour. Surgical intervention was prompted by a sustained and worrying rise in blood pressure and was carried out only after Mrs Ekoku had been convinced of the dangers of continuing with a normal delivery. She was bitterly disappointed at this turn of events. The baby weighed just over seven pounds and there were no apparent health problems apart from a minor eye irritation which developed shortly before their discharge home.

Jaruba was circumcised in accordance with his parents' cultural traditions at around seventeen days, an event which Mrs Ekoku could barely think about and which seemed somehow to deepen her own birth wound.

One can think that in the African context this tradition might carry with it a weight born of necessity in terms of hygiene, prevention of infection and possibly sexual codes, but, far from home, there were signs of some misgivings. Arrangements for the operation were quite complicated and this seemed to be not only to do with finding an appropriate person to carry it out, but also a reflection of some ambivalence about it which I heard played out in a telephone conversation. Moreover, Mrs Ekoku told me about the circumcision in a hesitant way which left me in little doubt that my opinion was being sought. This may well have been to do with ideas about what I, as a white person, might make of their actions, but it also seemed to represent the way in which these parents were caught up in ongoing negotiations for themselves around racial and cultural identity. In this sense, the decision about circumcision takes on another dimension, that of confirming and validating them in their difference, and may thus involve at a deep level a potentially radical and threatening appraisal of long-held beliefs, ideas and obligations.

The first recorded observation showed Jaruba already meeting the world more than half-way. He was clearly eliciting an affectionate response from his father who held him virtually throughout. I noted that already he seemed alert to his environment including sounds both within and outside the room and also that he had begun to develop an ability to tolerate potentially insecure states, for example, a persistently poorly supported head. Mr Ekoku beamed at his son and at me as he told me, 'This is a very hungry boy' and went on to describe the baby's determination to find and hold on to the breast, feeding with gusto.

This raised important questions about how the capacities which Jaruba exhibited came to be acquired, in particular the interplay between constitutional factors and the pre- and peri-natal experience. It is, of course, impossible to know whether by the moment of birth Jaruba already had a sense, based on the fluctuations in mother's ability to nourish herself and possibly also to give space in her mind to her own needs and her baby's existence, that he would have to strive to make his presence felt and to make the most of what was available to him. What became very clear as the observation progressed, was the way in which the circumstances of his conception and its consequences in terms of poverty, isolation and perilous insecurity, which were inextricably linked with the marginalisation of minority status, had an impact on his development. The importance of Jaruba's strong capacity for survival became apparent as this infant struggled to engage his mother, to manage her absences and to negotiate his way in the world.

GROWING UP

It was painfully apparent quite early on that the relationship between Jaruba and his mother was in some difficulty. There was a sense that mother felt held hostage by her son; she talked early on of feeling closed in and in response set out on long and exhausting treks around the streets in all weathers. The darkened and impoverished room which seemed to be the focal point of the house was furnished in a just-adequate, utility fashion with items belonging to other people, whilst much of what belonged to the couple remained in boxes; the drawn curtains and the locked doors juxtaposed with photographs of sunnier times, sunnier climes and bright wedding smiles hanging on the walls were a tangible expression of her sense of siege, alienation and inner depletion, at odds with the hopes and expectations of marriage and family life. Moreover, Mrs Ekoku's behaviour had a markedly more disturbed quality to it than what Margot Waddell (1987: 5) describes as 'the kind of depression which seems to follow naturally from the experience of giving birth, often extending into the first few weeks and sometimes months'.

Jaruba's needs seemed to be experienced as increasingly anxiety-provoking and mother responded to her inability to bear his dependency with denial and flight interspersed with fleeting and fearfully poignant moments of closeness and attunement. The following extract from the fifth observation is one of a number of illustrations of this.

Mrs Ekoku chats to me as she busily prepares for Jaruba's bath time. She begins to undress him, saying 'He really doesn't like this'; within seconds of removing his arm from the sleeve of the babygro he begins to cry and this escalates to a mixture of a cry and a yell. It seems that his whole body is involved in the crying, his torso is stiff, his arms shaking frantically, fists still clenched, his stiff legs kicking and jerking.

His face is screwed up and his brow furrowed. I ask Mrs Ekoku if there are tears on Jaruba's face and she replies brightly, 'Oh yes, come over and see.' The final item to be removed is his nappy and as she walks away to deposit this in the bin Jaruba seems to be in absolute despair, his frantic movements becoming more exaggerated and his cries louder.

Mrs Ekoku carries on her conversation with me though I can recall little of what is said and I am aware of a to-ing and fro-ing between what seems to be a complete disconnection (no eye contact or comforting gestures) and being in touch as she talks soothingly and sympathetically to him, using a pet name, telling him he will be dressed soon.... There is relief all round it seems when he is lifted from the bath and a precious few moments follow when Mrs Ekoku massages oil into his body and both look as if they are connected in their enjoyment.

When Jaruba was around six weeks of age I learned that he was no longer being breast-fed because, as Mrs Ekoku described it, she felt unable to fill him – he was always hungry and always wanting to be at the breast. The transition to bottle-feeding was talked about pragmatically, though I had a sense that at a deeper level Mrs Ekoku had experienced her baby's demands as draining the life from her. She became increasingly preoccupied with some academic work which she had started before her pregnancy and on more than one occasion I arrived to find her seated at her desk, positioned in a way which literally turned her back on Jaruba who lay awake, unblinking and unacknowledged on the sofa behind her.

This preoccupation later shifted to that of finding paid employment and she obtained a full-time post some considerable distance away which, with travel, meant at least a twelve-hour day and predictably left her feeling exhausted. In response to this state of affairs she eventually found work closer to home, yet shortly afterwards she acquired an additional job which involved working three nights each week. Effectively, this took her away from home for longer periods than before and whilst this could have, in part, been connected with financial pressures, it became evident that Mrs Ekoku would also take on unpaid additional commitments seemingly regardless of the impact on her personal resources or her family life.

It did seem that any sign of need in Jaruba led to his mother distancing him even further, as illustrated by the following material from the eighteenth observation when Jaruba was just under twelve months old.

> Mrs Ekoku begins to be able to talk in a less agitated way about life in general and Jaruba becomes increasingly unsettled as she attempts to shift him from her lap. When he starts to whimper again she moves him towards the opposite end of the sofa from her and offers a pot of fromage frais; he manages about three spoons before losing interest whimpering and holding out his arms to her. She turns him so that he can see the TV and picks up again on her earlier comments to me about her concerns about Jaruba's childminder.

This possibly desperate need to absent herself from the unbearably intimate encounters with her baby evoked very powerful feelings of despair and disapproval both in myself as observer and within the seminar group, particularly when concerns began to emerge about childminding arrangements.

The seminar setting began to feel at times a less than comfortable or satisfactory place in which to reflect on those aspects of Mrs Ekoku's temperament and personality which seemed to create particular difficulties for her as an individual and as a mother. To some extent this was to do with a growing awareness within the group of the complexities and limitations of the essentially white, Eurocentric theoretical and ideological framework within which we were thinking about what was being observed, and our genuine misgivings about the pervasiveness and determinism of the particular socio-cultural contexts within which we had developed as individuals and which we shared in unspoken ways in group interactions.

Mrs Ekoku, on several occasions, talked movingly about how things would be different were she at home in Africa, the automatic expectation of Jaruba's grandmothers being that they would undertake responsibility for his care whilst his mother resumed her career and contribution to the family income. It became increasingly apparent to me that the socio–cultural constructions to which this mother had been exposed did not have at their heart a notion of the exclusivity or specialness of the relationship between birth mother and baby which seems so firmly rooted, even idealised, in contemporary Western approaches to child-rearing. In Mrs Ekoku's culture of origin, the emphasis was placed on collective responsibility for meeting the infant's needs, including the need for what we might term 'mother love'. Indeed, many of those working across cultures in refugee organisations and counselling services have pointed to the erroneous application of what has been termed 'the cult of the individual'. The conceptualisation of needs and the pursuit of happiness and security in crudely individualistic terms appears to belong almost entirely to contemporary Western cultures and such ideas are in essence alien to many of different cultural background.

In the normal course of events in her country of origin, Mrs Ekoku would not expect to be mothering a child until she became a grandmother. This puts a different perspective on her capacity for containment and the meeting of her baby's needs, at this stage in her life, or even whether there could be a real sense that this is something she should be doing. She longed for her own mother to be with her just as many Western mothers would but with the added connotation that her mother and her husband's mother both had a rightful place in looking after baby Jaruba.

This issue of mothering highlights in an important way the inadequacy of employing an over-simplistic juxtaposition of theoretical approaches and cultural perspectives in order to understand and explain complex behaviours. We need to question the extent to which the sense of siege and inner depletion stemmed from the fears which her baby's helplessness evoked and amplified in Mrs Ekoku, putting her harshly in touch with her own feelings of emptiness. We know that such feelings, accompanied by aloneness and isolation, are not uncommon for many mothers, and we can perhaps draw some parallels with the impact of geographical and social mobility in the British context, specifically the fragmentation of family and community ties and communal obligations. But for Mrs Ekoku there was the overlay of an experience also of being alienated from the taken-for-granted, comfortably familiar codes of a mainstream culture which could only heighten her sense of being unheld and unbelonging, cut adrift from her cultural roots and the practical support of an extended family network.

Viewed in this light, perhaps it is unsurprising that Mrs Ekoku catches hold of her intellectual abilities as an emotional life-raft and translates good-enough mothering into material provision. Indeed, there is an intelligibility to her actions of turning to her professional life and the need to provide tangibly and concretely for her child if this is located in an adherence to the cultural codes and expectations within which she herself had been raised. This became problematic, of course, when transposed to a different cultural context where there were no grandmothers to call upon and where she and her husband failed to find satisfactory alternative carers.

Whatever its origin in terms of the precise nature–nurture interplay, Mrs Ekoku's limited capacity for containment, that is, the difficulties she seemed to have in keeping her baby in her mind and meeting his dependency needs in any consistent way, did have a profound impact on Jaruba's development. I, as observer, became filled with preoccupations about the range of adversities facing this child which could be conceptualised as the observer to an extent operating as a container of infantile anxieties at a time when mother seemed to be unable to do so.

With each successive observation there was growing evidence of a denial on the part of both parents that Jaruba was a real baby with a baby's needs, a denial of his human-ness and even, at times, of his existence. It was extremely difficult as an observer to bear the emotional distress evoked in me whilst simultaneously struggling to sustain a thoughtful, non-judgemental frame of mind. There was little sense of Jaruba reaching his milestones at his own pace, rather he lurched towards them with metaphorically gritted teeth. There were frequent references in my observations to how grown up he appeared and to both parents' demands for demonstrations of his independence.

The seminar group struggled with descriptions of Jaruba as animal-like, or as making raw, primitive sounds, or as behaving in a savage way. These words, which we would have felt relatively at ease using in relation to an infant of similar cultural background, became imbued in this cultural context with a prickliness, even dangerousness, which left us immobilised in our explorations of this infant's experience and puzzled as to why we should have responded in this particular way. Despite the personal impact of the following sequence, which resonated within the seminar setting, I found myself seeking alternative, culturally sensitive or rather 'correct' explanations to my description of Jaruba being treated much as one would a pet, even questioning whether I 'really' saw and felt what I did see and feel.

Mrs E says she will fetch cake for Jaruba . . . she spreads newspaper on the floor, puts the plate on the paper, calls Jaruba over and sits him on it. I am struck immediately by how this would seem more in keeping with caring for an animal, a messy puppy and I find the scene distressing to observe as he flips over a piece of cake, picks up a large crumb and discards it. He just sits momentarily on the paper . . . my heart goes out to him.

My reflections on this event struck me as going beyond a healthy questioning of values and attitudes and was uncomfortably redolent of the inversely racist approaches which allow for child maltreatment to continue on the basis of some loosely formed ideas about the legitimation of certain behaviours by their cultural context.

The seminar's unease, at least in part, stemmed from mixed feelings about the appropriateness or validity of material about a black child and his family being processed by a white observer within a white seminar group reliant on theoretical perspectives informed by observations (largely) of white children.

I am mindful here of studies of black family life which have rightly in recent years been criticised at a number of levels. The dubious assumptions on which research protocols have been based, the fundamental flaws in methodology and the misrepresentation of data have fostered a view of black family life as essentially pathological and dysfunctional. Algea Harrison (1988: 220) notes how the failure to view the parenting style of black mothers from the perspective of their own culture has produced data which is highly critical of their behaviour, apparently finding it detrimental to sex-role socialisation, cognitive development and a variety of personality traits in black children.

The role of black males as fathers has also been a controversial research area, with investigations seemingly more concerned with effects of father absence than presence and Harrison (1988: 219) argues that there has been a failure to acknowledge the impact of the wider black community, culture differences in role prescriptions, and the importance of kinship systems. Indeed, in this observation I am, for quite a while, referring to Mr Ekoku as a shadowy figure, though it eventually comes to light that he undertakes the bulk of the childcare responsibility outside his working hours.

Clearly it is important to challenge hyper-critical and ill-informed judgements about particular cultural norms and parenting styles. However, the key issue which infant observation generally demonstrates, and which was striking in this particular observation, is how a specific cultural context impacts on an infant's development, especially when the networks which hold and sustain the individual in the culture of origin are not transferable to a different set of cultural circumstances. The problem, which became increasingly evident as the observation progressed, is how to think and learn about difference in ways which are truthful and sensitive when such powerful feelings are evoked. How are we to understand the impact upon infants of the child-rearing priorities, attitudes and patterns of behaviour which have developed out of the exigencies of the unique economic, racial and cultural circumstances in which ethnic minority families live and have lived? Moreover, what actually happens to infants when constructions on, and capacities for parenting, which are born of one cultural context are at odds with what is sustainable in another?

As Jaruba approached one year of age a sequence was recorded which vividly illustrated his depression, withdrawal and perhaps near collapse alongside his mother's reliance on distancing and what appeared to be the use of perpetual motion as a coping mechanism, as described by Bick (1987: 115).

> Mrs Ekoku bundles the pushchair into the flat... swiftly sets about taking Jaruba from the pram, removing her own coat and talking all the while about how hectic life is ... Jaruba is sitting quite still, mouth open. He is lifted from the pushchair, his face immobile, expression largely unchanged even when the pushchair, weighed down by the bags hanging from the handles, tips over. His coat is taken off in a rather perfunctory fashion and he is left momentarily standing in the hall, looking about him, shell-shocked, the almost silent beginnings of a whimper.

This was followed by a painful sequence with Jaruba serially displaced as he attempted to connect with his mother who offered a range of food and drink in place of her self, unable it seemed to pay him real attention. In this same observation my discomfort reached a peak when Mrs Ekoku began to reveal, for the first time, her anxieties about both Jaruba's former and current childminders. She described how with one minder she found Jaruba coiled up in a corner every time she collected him and how he flinched when she reached out to pick him up. This account of events and my response to it was further complicated by the rather detached style in which the information was delivered and by the fact that it was the black minders who were perceived to be inferior to the white minders. Whilst to an extent there appeared to be some evidential basis for this view, it raised questions about the significance of my own whiteness in this context, and the rejection of blackness with its correlative inferiority in relation to identity and self-concept in black individuals, which a number of researchers have documented (Maxime 1993: 96). What was most striking, however, was the way in which the adversities faced by this family impelled Mr and Mrs Ekoku towards an increasingly unrealistic requirement that their baby be independent, which in truth meant that he be non-dependent; which allowed them to leave their son with people whom they perceived as unsatisfactory.

This is an important distinction because at its heart is the difference between, on the one hand, a gradual and sequential development of the ability to be securely separate and self-containing (independence proper) and, on the other, a state of sink or swim adversity where feelings of dependency are not merely denied but cannot be recognised or acknowledged as having an existence (non-dependence). One can observe this *in extremis* in those who have experienced traumatic and/or, serial dislocations such as abandonment and repeated breakdowns in fostering or adoptive arrangements, a prevailing feature being the sense that all hope of dependency needs being met has been abandoned.

With regard to Jaruba, neither parent seemed able to think about independence arising out of dependency needs being met and he was expected at times to cope with situations of real torment. It was not difficult to imagine, for instance, the maelstrom of jealousy, rage and confusion into which Jaruba was catapulted when his mother picked up another child rather than him immediately on her return from work. His need to be gathered up by her following her absence seemed to be interpreted by Mrs Ekoku as evidence of some sort of failing in him, a negative personality trait, and she responded with an almost scornful disapproval. One wonders also whether something rather more complicated was being played out around rivalry and helplessness, possibly related to Mrs Ekoku's personal experiences of having to share parental figures and of a range of displacements, prejudices and preferments to which she may have been exposed because of the colour of her skin, her cultural or her tribal background.

In a rare account which Mrs Ekoku gave of aspects of her earlier life there were hints of possible difficulties around the meaning of independence as illustrated by the following excerpt when Jaruba was around fourteen months old.

> Mrs Ekoku goes on to talk about her hopes and intentions with regard to Jaruba's upbringing commenting that she wants him to be independent not 'spoiled' and over-dependent as she was . . . she tells me of her own childhood experiences, saying that right up until she left Africa she had no idea how to handle her money, buy her own clothes and she places this squarely at her father's door. Consequently when she first arrived in Germany, life was extremely difficult; she felt very homesick and totally at sea in terms of running her life, particularly her finances. She recalls that when things got really bad her father would arrange an air ticket for her to return home even for a weekend . . .

Mrs Ekoku's 'spoiling' seemed in her mind to be about parental failure to make her self-reliant thus leaving her exposed to a terrible, painful, internal state of inadequacy and unpreparedness for the adult world far from home. This experience did not seem to have been processed in a way which could be helpful to her son, rather it had become translated into a determination to make him independent, as if this is something one learns to do as distinct from to be. There was also something telling about the way in which education appears to have been grasped as a means not only of coping with difficult circumstances but, more significantly, as a way of escaping and/or growing out of her emotional predicament, that is, a utilisation of intellectual building blocks as a replacement or substitute for the kind of emotional knowledge which is required for progression towards maturity and which is born of dependency needs being adequately met.

This raised many questions about the interplay between individual personality traits, parental needs and cultural context in relation to the premium which seemed to be placed on the notion of independence however this might be understood. Was Mrs Ekoku describing a disturbing combination of under- and over-protective parenting? Was she telling me something about familial and cultural norms to do with who manages money and makes practical provision for members of the household? Was she letting me know about an experience of apparent independence which feels brittle and precarious?

Can this fierce independence and commitment to educational achievement be understood in other ways from a different cultural perspective? Does the importance attached to growing up quickly at whatever cost, in terms of dependency needs, or however insubstantial such independence or rather non-dependence might be, make sense in the context of the cultural and child-rearing patterns which these parents have experienced? Is this but one dimension of what Nobles, in his in his study of African-American families (1988: 49) describes as 'the unique child-rearing techniques which seem to be geared to prepare the child for a particular kind of existence in a hostile racial environment'.

We need to think about how patterns of behaviour which might be deemed maladaptive in one environment might in fact be adaptive in another, for example, the context of dealing day by day with attributions of inferiority and oppression born of a history of tribal conflict, slavery, contemporary nationalism and global racism.

The pseudo-independence which Jaruba actually acquired was concretely manifested in the striking bow shape of his legs. Mrs Ekoku connected this at an intellectual level, with him prematurely bearing his weight on his legs. She candidly acknowledged a causal link between the pressure Jaruba had been under from both parents to walk early and what had happened to his legs. However, there appeared to be no place in her mind for a consideration of how inappropriate such actions might have been, or how Jaruba might have experienced the mismatch between what was required of him and what he was actually capable of. It is perhaps telling that one of the most 'intimate' encounters recorded in the observation material between mother and son took place when Jaruba was in his mother's perception, at his most independent – taking his weight on his own two feet and only lightly supported by his mother's hands, the precariousness of which stirred considerable anxiety in the observer.

MOVING ON

As Jaruba and the observation entered the second year of life, the profound lack of containment to which he was exposed seemed set to continue unabated. In addition to mother's prolonged absences and the difficulties she seemed to experience in opening herself up to her son when she returned, there were a series of abrupt endings to unsatisfactory childminding arrangements to be contended with.

Jaruba had fairly frequent bouts of ill-health – chest and skin complaints, viruses and recurring diarrhoea which according to his mother cleared up at the weekend, a state of affairs she attributed to sloppy standards of hygiene at the childminder's. The observation recordings were peppered with accounts of Jaruba's behaviour which may be thought of as indicative of faulty development of the primal skin function as described by Bick (1987: 115) and to which I have already alluded.

There was considerable evidence of the operation of second skin mechanisms from the earliest displays of pseudo-independence in both mother and infant to Jaruba's marked utilisation in later months of a range of surfaces, physical activity and audio-visual sensory experience. The extent and degrees of physicality exhibited by Jaruba were striking features of this observation and seemed to have their counterpart in Mrs Ekoku's relentlessly hectic lifestyle. When Jaruba was not climbing, bouncing, falling, squealing or eating, he tended to slip into a forlorn, aimless state unless held by the TV screen or some other potentially containing presence including, occasionally, my lap. In similar vein, during holidays from work, when Mrs Ekoku was deprived of the demands and trappings of her status as a professional working woman, she seemed to sink into a routine of sleeping during the day and watching TV in a darkened room, the world beyond the flat shut out by the drawn curtains and an air of lifelessness prevailing.

The TV figured prominently throughout the observation period and there were many references in the material to its presence almost as a third party with which both Jaruba and mother frequently engaged. It soon became apparent that Jaruba's relationship with the screen represented something other than a healthy captivation with moving images, and I have selected one of many observed sequences as an illustration.

Jaruba wanders into the room quite slowly, his body seems to be sighing; he hesitates, moves towards the toy corner, as usual via the TV. He is groaning with his body and his voice, not able to engage with anything in particular though there are intermittent periods of focused concentration on the TV screen. I have a sense that Mrs Ekoku is rapidly becoming irritated by his behaviour. She offers a drink which he doesn't want and then a dummy which momentarily seems to satisfy him. . . . He wanders, rather grumbly and aimless over to the TV, places the dummy teat against the screen then strikes the screen once or twice, not heavily, with the dummy – he seems to be listening to the hollow sound which is emitted. . . . Jaruba is offered a bottle, he takes hold of it but almost instantaneously lets it go and the milk dribbles on to the carpet. He picks it up once or twice more and the same thing happens. Mrs Ekoku seems oblivious to this, her attention returns to the TV and she remarks that she thinks she will fall asleep.

There was an enormous amount of material which served to illustrate not only the multifarious ways in which surfaces were employed but also the complexities involved in thinking about their significance in relation to second skin formation both within the broad context of infant development and the more specific one of race-culture connotations. Some of Jaruba's second skin defences seemed very evidently to operate as a means of defence in the face of real or perceived threats to his precarious inner state; this appeared to be reassuringly straightforward despite being painful to observe. For instance, the transition from childminder to home was almost always an uneasy one for Jaruba which he managed by touching his fingers together as he entered the room, adhering to pieces of furniture or, as in the following sequence:

Jaruba stands at the door to the lounge, his back against the frame; he looks sullen, perhaps anxious as he surveys the room making one or two grumbly sounds . . . he hesitates then slowly edges his way into the room, his back and the palms of both hands lightly against the wall.

There are, however, rather more complex sequences which are observed, some characterised by a marked incongruity, for example a simultaneous manifestation of both sturdiness and fragility in the way Jaruba conducted himself and others where an ostensibly intimate and primal skin-to-skin encounter appeared quite unpredictably to become imbued with a highly charged excitability, erotism and/or aggression. For instance in one observation:

Mother flops lengthways on the sofa, her dress falling above her knees exposing an expanse of flesh. Jaruba's attention returns to the TV and he does an odd little squatting dance which brings sexual connotations to my mind and seems to embarrass mother. He smiles, seems self-absorbed, then with a little sigh gets back in touch with his surroundings and climbs on to his mother. She is lying on her side and at first he settles himself into the curve of her body where he looks extremely comfortable held in the cradling dip of her waist rising to the hip. They

> both watch TV for a few moments then Jaruba launches a series of what seem to be rough grabbing-pulling movements as he grasps his way over his mother's body. He makes a grab for her earrings and then roughly tugs at her headscarf, loosening his grip and momentarily becoming gentler as she struggles to hold on to it . . . he then drops on to her upper body, half stroking, half grabbing her left breast.

Whilst second skin mechanisms helped Jaruba to manage a range of adversities there were obviously serious concerns about the extent to which they replaced the introjection of a real containing object, with consequences for his intellectual, emotional and personality development. In particular, he ran the risk of the development of a two-dimensional type of personality constructed from an adhesive mode of identification, where the processes of identification take place less in the service of growth and development but more as a way of defending against the reality of separation. Adhesive modes of identification are characterised by a carapace quality, the resulting sense of identity is fragile and based on imitation, mimicry and resemblance of the personality traits of others; in short, an identity is put on rather than taken in, formed from an adaptation to the dominant mode and prevailing fashions to which the individual is exposed at any given time.

This mode of functioning can sustain individuals for some time and, superficially, all can appear to be well. Problems arise when life events, for example an age-related separation such as leaving home for work or college, opens up the individual to the terrifying awareness of there being nothing of any substance inside.

There were indications of another aspect of Jaruba's personality when, in an observation characterised by a manic air of physicality, a sequence was recorded in which he bounced, jumped, bumped against and fell off a range of surfaces culminating in what seemed to be a sado-masochistic interlude, disturbing to me as observer and subsequently to the seminar group:

> With some encouragement from mother, Jaruba climbs up on the sofa and there is a fairly lengthy period of kissing, cuddling and snuggling; mother rubs her face into Jaruba's cheeks and they both squeal and giggle. She kisses him over and over again, holding him lengthways against her outstretched body, both arms wrapped around him in what seems to be a comfortable grip. He becomes very excited, working himself up into a near orgasmic pitch of squeals and then in a combination of mother letting go and Jaruba wriggling free he sinks back into the sofa settling behind her outstretched legs. The excitement persists and he sways his upper body repeatedly from side to side.

Later:

Mother holds Jaruba tightly on her knee ... his back against her chest and he struggles to get free. The struggle becomes quite violent, he jerks his head back and hits her hard on the jaw. She grins, rubs her hand against one side of her face still holding on to Jaruba with the other arm, his expression is glazed and I have the feeling that we are all momentarily suspended as I engage in my own struggle to think about what I have just seen.

This was a confusing episode not least for Jaruba, confronted by the incongruity of mother's grin in response to a forceful and meaningful blow and the possibility that some excitement was stirred in her by this violent attack. Further, his long-felt and frequently displayed need to be held tightly by her somehow became an unbearably oppressive experience from which he had to escape.

There was a further dimension to Jaruba's behaviour and interactions which seemed to be of related significance in terms of the frequency with which he came perilously close to hurting himself or actually was injured. His accident-proneness and the escalating danger of some of his activities were particularly prominent features towards the end of Jaruba's first year and continued into his second year of life; I did begin to wonder whether there might be a sado-masochistic quality to what was going on inside him. This may be attributable to a number of factors not least the possible significance of primitive and deep-seated anxieties, linked with a lack of internal resources and a consequent reliance on a false, omnipotent strength. There can be little doubt that Jaruba's tendency to find himself in positions where harm was imminent and seemingly inevitable was complex and multi-faceted but in one particular aspect there were hints of a somewhat dysfunctional kind of interaction taking place. Some typical examples follow:

> Within what seems to be seconds Jaruba lurches at my lap/hands, knocking the cup with the result that some of the hot tea splashes on his fingers. Mother rushes over, picks him up and carries him into the kitchen.

and again:

> Jaruba climbs on to the polished and sharp edged table and stands on it, something his mother does not seem to see ... later he goes back to the table and the accident which seems to be waiting to happen does happen and he falls, banging his head and letting out a wailing cry. Mother dashes to him, picks him up, holding him closely and cradling his head against her shoulder.

The common feature here is the outcome of the accidents; Jaruba is eventually in union with a previously unavailable mother, not through a straightforward expression of and response to his need but rather as a result of what struck me as a possibly perverse process of double-edged perilous excitation and self-injury.

The ramifications of being close for this mother and son are vividly apparent in the following sequence:

> Initially Jaruba is standing off from his mother, a sense of hostility and uncertainty around ... there is a brief interlude where they play in a rough and tumble sort of way, Jaruba held upside down. I am aware of smiling over at them, willing it to be a good experience, but Jaruba is not comfortable. He has a mixed expression of pleasure though not satisfaction and fear alongside apprehension. This looks like an activity which easily could get out of control and become rougher. There is a sense of aggressive tension, even violence beneath the surface; Jaruba appears to be glad of the physical contact but a safer experience might be preferable to him although one suspects that he might find straight-forward hugs and cuddles quite difficult to handle. I become aware of the smell of faeces on Jaruba. An image from another observation flashes into my mind – Jaruba fiercely struggling, his face contorted in hate as mother grips him hard, saying half-playfully, half-mockingly, 'You are my prisoner', whilst I sit, desperate to call a halt to what feels like a truly awful interlude.

There seemed to me little doubt that, at times, I was in close proximity to the perilous states of mind in which, as Rosenfeld (1982: 53) puts it, 'love and hate impulses and good and bad objects cannot be kept apart resulting in confusion and anxiety such that the whole self is felt to be in danger of being destroyed'.

It is important to keep in mind that love and hate ordinarily coincide in the development of emotional life and attachment to others, especially in infancy. Indeed, it is precisely in relation to such states of confusion and conflictual anxiety in her baby that the mother's capacity for containment is so critical to the attribution of meaning to and thus the proper integration of experience. I have already drawn attention to Bion's view (1988: 37) of the adverse impact upon the infant when projections are not contained and transformed by maternal reverie. In these circumstances the process of projective identification can be seen to have failed in its aim of communication and becomes instead what Miller (1992: 124) has described as a forceful evacuation giving rise to fragmentation of the self and confusion between self and object.

Whilst it is evident that the concept of infantile hate can be problematic, particularly so from a lay perspective, the possibility that mothers experience real hate impulses towards their babies seems even more difficult to contemplate. In characteristically perspicacious and unsentimental fashion, Winnicott (1958: 202), acknowledges the reality and the power of a mother's love but also lists reasons why a mother hates her baby pointing out that:

> A mother has to be able to tolerate hating her baby without doing anything about it. She cannot express it to him. If, for fear of what she may do, she cannot hate appropriately when hurt by her child she must fall back on masochism. . . . The most remarkable thing about a mother is her ability to be hurt so much by her baby and to hate so much without paying the child out, and her ability to wait for rewards that may or may not come at a later date.

The emotional management of hate has also to be understood in context, specifically in regard to the interplay between hate as experienced in the internal world and hate as a feature of external reality which, in this particular observation, included issues of racial identity and racial oppression. As her theories about the nature of the internal mental life of individuals evolved, Melanie Klein drew attention many times to the powerful influence which external circumstances can have on shaping the internal world. Of particular relevance here is the way in which external reality is used to test internal reality with possible consequences when this process is not one of reciprocal modulation in the light of affirming experience, but one of distortion and falsehood.

In her therapeutic work with black children, Maxime (1993: 99) acknowledges the importance of Klein's contribution to assisting the understanding of racial identity development in young children and, indeed, in offering a possible explanation for the incidence of identity crisis and self-hatred. She states:

> Klein emphasised that a young child's perception of external reality and external objects is perpetually influenced and coloured by his or her experiences. She stressed that it was impossible to separate the outer and inner realities completely as they overlapped. The area of Klein's work which is of importance is that in which she highlights a child's inexperience of a certain negative external reality and the frustration the child experiences as it is beyond his or her comprehension. Thus a child's inexperience in integrating the outer and inner realities stands unprotected against this interaction and projects that rage onto his or her external objects while internalising the same object in all its terror and fearfulness.
>
> (Maxime 1993: 99)

If one applies this to the personality development of black children then it immediately becomes apparent that there is potential for hate impulses to be amplified in an external world where bigotry, race hate and systematic discrimination may be an everyday experience. Persecutory and paranoid anxieties can thus be projected into an environment where they thrive rather than undergo modification and where re-introjection in gross and exaggerated forms occurs. This environment is, of course, the mother's mind in the first instance and, for a black woman in a white host culture, there may be the residues of the experience of the systematic attribution of inferiority, badness and a range of other negative connotations to black-ness. Moreover, I have come to question whether there is a white aspect of herself in some black mothers' minds whose idealised phantasy baby is white and who have to bring this together with the reality of a baby whose blackness serves as a repository for many of the ills of white society.

In my view, all of this has potentially grave consequences for the development of identity in black people because of the corrosiveness of being split off and set apart in one's difference. This not only militates against integration in each individual but has its counterpart in the communities and social systems within which individuals live and where this issue of integration has long occupied those concerned with race relations.

COMING THROUGH

As I observed the hardships which Jaruba and his parents endured yet also witnessed the strivings of this infant to make his way in the world, at times, it seemed, against all odds, I began to wonder about the extent to which Jaruba might be falling short in his developmental potential. I had to bear not only the evidence of the impact of the lack of containment, but also speculations about what sort of developmental path he might have taken had there been less suffering for him to contend with, and what had been lost on the way. Such reflections put me in touch with what was lacking in terms of maternal reverie and what was lost between this mother and son. There were also a range of projections around parental guilt and inadequacy to be coped with, heightened by my identification with baby Jaruba and my personal circumstances as the mother of a young baby. The processing of material within the containing environment of the seminar group was critical in sustaining me in the observer role and also in identifying those pockets of hope and resilience which seemed so elusive early on. In this respect, one could reflect on what kind of influence the presence of black colleagues might have had on the identification and exploration of positive trends.

What became clear as the second year of the observation progressed was that Jaruba was not crushed by the adversities which had been evident throughout, and his capacity for holding on to himself, glimpsed in the early days, seemed to remain largely undiminished. One of Jaruba's most striking features was his persistence, he just didn't give up and was observed on a number of occasions to have remarkable success in eventually gaining what he needed, albeit sometimes assisted by the observer's presence or by mother being gathered in some other way, for example, through a telephone call from her husband.

Jaruba also proved to be adept at securing containing experiences, swiftly recognising and taking up opportunities to be held. He made the most of times when mother was able to be available to him, when he could, actually or symbolically, find a place for himself on a lap and there was growing evidence of an ability to capitalise on his positive childminding experiences when they occurred and the presence of an observer. He tended to seek out symbolic containers which seemed to assist him in giving of himself and in turn would sometimes enable his mother to give of herself as illustrated by this sequence:

> Jaruba finds a little space for himself between the coffee table and an armchair and settles there for a few moments . . . he seems to be looking for something which I realise is the orange which mother gave to him. He can't quite get hold of it. He looks over to mother, an open expression on his face, and she lifts him gently over the coffee table and gives him a hug . . . Jaruba is full of smiles.

As he grew older, Jaruba's use of play to communicate, make sense of or master his experience, came into its own, for instance in an observation where he had been struggling to be in a threesome with mother and a neighbour's child, the following sequence occurred:

> Jaruba slips into a triangular space created by the coffee table being placed in a particular way next to the sofa arm. He seems comfortable in this space, his sullen rather preoccupied air finally lifts. . . . Jaruba decides he wants to be out of the triangle and makes several attempts to extricate himself. . . . I am struck by his patience, his sturdiness and his ingenuity as he makes a series of manoeuvres . . .

There are many occasions when his play appears to be an acting out of an internal experience, for example, in one observation where he is serially pulled towards and pushed away from his mother he engages in play with a door, repetitively pulling it to and fro. In another observation he holds 'in suspension' a piece of bread which mother has offered in response to him wanting to be taken back into her arms. He drops the bread which seemed, as it were in place of mother, and he forgets it in what appeared to be a vivid expression of an experience of being dropped, cast out of mind and forgotten.

At around eighteen months of age there were consistent signs that things were beginning to improve. Life for both Jaruba and his mother seemed fuller, more three-dimensional and varied. There appeared to be genuine moments of pleasure in each other's company and Mrs Ekoku expressed for the first time a sense of her significance to her son:

Mrs Ekoku says that she is beginning to realise how Jaruba might miss her and goes on to describe a recent party where Jaruba stayed awake long after the other children had gone to sleep in order to see her when she returned at 9.00 p.m. She had been told that he would not settle until she came and seems quite taken by this discovery.

Jaruba's expanding vocabulary appeared to be immensely important in terms of allowing him to have a dialogue with his parents which was valued and which moved his relationship with them on to a different plane. Interestingly, his play became increasingly focused on making contact and opening up communication and there was a corresponding diminution of the rather random, aimless quality which had previously been observed.

Within the seminar setting there was much interest in the factors which had brought about what appeared to be a turning point. It was noted that some of the internal insecurities and perceived external threats which drove the couple to Britain, seemed to have lost some of their potency. We wondered whether Mrs Ekoku's sparkle could be attributed to a shift in her relationship with her husband or were we perhaps seeing a mother only just beginning to recover from the birth of her son?

Certainly there is no shortage of evidence of the potentially adverse effects of maternal depression, even in its milder manifestations, on the quality of attachment. Jane Corrigan's recent work (1992), for instance, has drawn attention to the importance of the baby's smiling response and how the absence of this combined with the infant's neediness is particularly difficult for depressed mothers to bear. This means, of course, that the critical first few weeks following birth can be especially taxing before a smiling response can develop in the baby and when the mother herself may be experiencing unprecedented degrees of vulnerability and neediness. It did seem very evident in this observation that the more Jaruba was able to give of himself, particularly with regard to managing the daily, energy-sapping and thankless routines of life, the more relaxed his mother was able to become and there was a growing sense that she began to feel loved rather than drained by him.

One of the most significant events in the life of the Ekoku family during the observation and one which I rather conspicuously overlooked was a visit from a relative from Africa, Mr Ekoku's brother. The immediately positive effects of this seemed somewhat disproportionate to my sensibilities and I had assumed that his presence had a less significant impact than on reflection proved to be the case. Both Mr and Mrs Ekoku were lit up by his being with them, by news of family happenings and by the concrete representations of home in the form of spices and delicacies which accompanied him.

The ordinary way in which Mrs Ekoku told me of his suggestion that Jaruba might live for a while with the family in Africa left me stunned and I was perplexed by what seemed to be her embarrassment that she did not feel able to let him go. I thought of Jaruba's extended family as strangers and could not seriously entertain the thought that such a move might even be contemplated. With some difficulty I came to recognise that I was attempting to make intelligible a set of circumstances from a perspective on family life that was completely at odds with their own and becoming extremely judgemental in the process.

Niara Sudarkasa (1988: 30) argues forcefully that black families must be understood as institutions with historical traditions which set them apart as alternative formations that are neither identical to nor patho- logical variants of family structures found among other groups. For instance, the most far-reaching difference between African and European families stems, she suggests, from their differential emphasis on con- sanguinity (blood ties) and conjugality (the affinal kinship created between spouses). In Africa, unlike in Europe, in many critical areas of family life, the consanguineal core group rather than the conjugal pair has been paramount.

CONCLUDING THOUGHTS

The experience of infant observation is an extraordinarily rich and compel- ling one. But more than this, as a learning method which is rigorous and painstaking it holds out real promise of taking us forward in our thinking about difference and how it impacts on us all.

There is much to be gained from increasing our awareness and under- standing of racial and cultural variations, perceptions and experiences. We need to be purposeful in opening up the experience of infant observation in a way which reflects the reality of the multi-racial and multi-cultural society in which we live in Britain. This means thinking positively and sensitively about how same-race and trans-race cultural observations are negotiated and how recorded material is properly processed. The issue of consent, for example, has an added dimension where there are obvious power differentials between observer and observed. Seminar groups which are exclusively white or have in attendance one black colleague are plainly less than satisfactory regardless of the ethnic origin of the infant being observed if we really wish to broaden our understanding of how develop- ment might be shaped. It can be a salutary experience to learn of the incredulity expressed by other nationalities at some of the orthodox British child-rearing practices of which sleeping arrangements and toilet training are common examples.

In my view, observation offers the possibility of studying 'differentness' in ways which need not be characterised by schism, fear and opprobrium. And finally, returning to the plight of the silver shilling, the tale ends when he eventually finds his way into the hands of a traveller from his country of origin. The traveller's recognition of him, not as a false coin but as a 'good honest shilling' in a different world validates his 'differentness', restores him and makes him 'righted at last'.

REFERENCES

Andersen, Hans Christian (1983) *Complete Stories*, translated by H. C. Dulcken, London: Chancellor Press (first published 1889).

Banks, J. and Grambs, J. (1972) *Black Self Concept*, New York: McGraw-Hill.

Bick, E. (1987) 'The experience of skin in early object relations', in M. Harris Williams (ed.) *The Collected Papers of Martha Harris and Esther Bick*, Strath Tay, Perthshire: Clunie Press (first published 1970).

Bion, W. R. (1984) *Second Thoughts*, London: Karnac Books/Maresfield Library (first published by Heinemann 1967).

Bion, W. R. (1988) *Learning from Experience*, London: Maresfield (first published by Heinemann 1962).

Corrigan, Dr J. (1992) 'Post-natal depression and adverse effects on infancy', unpublished paper, Winnicott Research Unit.

Divine, D. (1984) 'Black children in care', *Caribbean Times*, 5 March.

Harris, M. (1987) 'Some notes on maternal containment in good enough mothering', in M. Harris Williams (ed.) *The Collected Papers of Martha Harris and Esther Bick*, Strath Tay, Perthshire: Clunie Press (first published 1970).

Harrison, A. O. (1988) 'Attitudes towards procreation among black adults', in H. P. McAdoo (ed.) *Black Families*, 2nd edn, London: Sage Publications.

High, H. (1992) 'Impediments to the development of attachment', *Psychoanalytic Psychotherapy*, 6, 2: 107–20.

Klein, M. (1932) *The Psycho-Analysis of Children*, London: Hogarth Press and the Institute of Psycho-Analysis.

Klein, M. (1988) *Love, Guilt and Reparation and Other Works 1921–1945*, London: Virago.

Maxime, J. E. (1993) 'The therapeutic importance of racial identity in working with black children who hate', in V. Varma (ed.) *How and Why Children Hate*, London: Jessica Kingsley.

Miller, L. (1992) 'The difficulty of establishing a space for thinking in the therapy of a 7-year-old girl', *Journal of Psychoanalytic Psychotherapy*, 6, 2: 121–135.

Nobles, W. W. (1988) 'African-American family life: an instrument of culture', in H. P. McAdoo (ed.) *Black Families*, London: Sage Publications.

Piontelli, A. (1989) 'A study on twins before and after birth', *International Review of Psycho-analysis*, 16, 4: 413–426.

Rosenfeld, H. A. (1982) *Psychotic States: A Psychoanalytic Approach*, London: Karnac Books/Maresfield Reprints (first published 1950).

Small, J. (1982) 'Black children in care: good practice guide (transracial placements)', unpublished paper presented to New Black Families Unit.

Sudarkasa, N. (1988) 'Interpreting the African heritage in Afro-American family organisation', in H. P. McAdoo (ed.) *Black Families*, London: Sage Publications.

Waddell, M. (1987) 'Infantile development: Kleinian and post-Kleinian theory, infant observational practice', unpublished Tavistock Clinic Paper No. 55.

Waddell, M. (1992) 'Adolescence and modes of identification', unpublished paper.

Winnicott, D. W. (1958) 'Hate in the countertransference', in *Collected Papers: Through Paediatrics to Psycho-analysis*, London: Tavistock (first published 1947).

Part II

Theoretical developments

Introduction

Susan Reid

The child psychoanalytic tradition attaches particular importance to the contribution to subsequent development of the earliest experiences of life, including experiences *in utero*. It has for some years been argued that findings about the emotional and unconscious life of infancy, generated by retrospective clinical reconstruction in psychotherapy and psychoanalysis with children and adults, could usefully be complemented by first-hand observation of infants. Such observation has played a significant, though until recently subordinate, role in the development of psychoanalytic ideas (Freud 1920; Klein 1952; Winnicott 1958; Bick 1964; Harris 1987).

More recent writers, for example Piontelli (1986, 1987, 1992) and Miller *et al.* (1989), have sought to demonstrate, using empirical observational evidence, how this contribution could be enhanced.

The chapters in this section continue in this tradition. The theoretical developments each author details are illustrated by excerpts from actual infant observations. This allows the reader the possibility of a more inter-active reading of the text; the excerpts let the reader follow the developments in each author's ideas and evaluate their conclusions. We believe that theoretical developments, illustrated in this way, stimulate the reader's own thinking and capacity to make associations to their work and life experiences. This parallels the suggestion (Chapter 1) that the practice of infant observation itself stimulates and supports the observer's own critical faculties. Agreement or disagreement with the theories postulated is therefore of secondary importance to their capacity to stimulate a lively response in the reader. The interweaving of infant observation material which has sparked a new idea into life allows the reader to share something of the process engaged in by each author.

Chapter 5, 'First light: knowing the infant as an actuality and as an idea', sits on the cusp of the first and second sections of this book and links with Isca Wittenberg's chapter on the explorations of the roles of observer, seminar group and seminar leader. Eric Rhode explores the conception of mind as a rationality, tracing his thinking through Melanie Klein's ideas about the evolution of the depressive position out of the paranoid-schizoid position (an historical developmental construction), to Bion's realisation that there is a constant oscillation between the two states throughout life. He suggests that the two positions and the threshold between them are logically anterior to stages of development. He draws from Wordsworth, Descartes and William Golding to illustrate his idea that, in psychoanalytic terms, 'our conjoined good objects are always thinking within us' from the very beginning and not just from birth. These ideas are linked with the function of the seminar leader attending to intuitions, which derive from the good objects and which potentially exist in every member of the seminar group. The seminar leader's capacity to tune in to the thinking good objects is enhanced by the very fact of not having been present at the actual observation. These ideas are illustrated by material from an infant observation. He describes the double responsibility of the seminar leader in supporting the commonsensical inclinations in the observer, essential in order to carry out the observations, whilst simultaneously attending to the 'intuitions' which give access to primary structures of the mind.

Chapter 6, 'Moments of discovery, times of learning', is the result of pioneering work which Alex Dubinsky and Olga Bazhenova began in Moscow. Their students took with enthusiasm to the new methodology, finding it a rich source of ideas which proved helpful when responding to the enormous need, in this rapidly changing society, for effective initiatives in planning mental health services.

Using illustrations provided by detailed observational material from two infant observations undertaken in Moscow, the authors explore, for both mother and infant, the role of *interest* in the manifestations of the other's mind, in encouraging development. This interest is described as essentially emotionally driven. The authors draw on the work of Vygotsky, Bion, Bick and Klein to support the view that, from the beginning of life after birth, the infant has a relation to mother which most significantly includes the mother's mind.

In Chapter 7, 'Thoughts on the containing process from the perspective of infant/mother relations', Pamela Berse Sorensen explores the concept of 'containment' and the 'containing process' with extraordinary clarity, drawing on material from infant observation and from clinical work.

Containment must be one of the most helpful concepts ever formulated; it finds frequent expression throughout this book. Bion in *Learning from Experience* (1962) described the container–contained relationships as the process by which one human being communicates with another. The *container* (often mother) is open to the communications, described as projections and projective identification from the infant. The *container* then contains the projections or communications (sometimes urgent, particularly in early infancy) by the process Bion described as *reverie* – a concept which Rhode utilises in his chapter. Providing the 'container' is in good enough emotional shape, she can then allow the baby's communications to resonate inside her so that they inform her subsequent responses. Containment used in this way implies holding on to, and not returning the feelings aroused, until some modifying work has been done. When this process fails, the mother either does not process the infant's communications at all, leaving the infant unrelieved, or worse, adds some emotional distress or confusion of her own, thereby making the infant feel much worse. There is a normative aspect to this, as Sorensen herself underlines. In any one day, any mother's capacities to 'contain' fluctuates, influenced by many factors such as other demands upon her attention or lack of sleep. It is only a cause for concern when there is long-term inadequate containment or excessive projection into the infant, by those who would normally be expected to be containing (see particularly Chapters 4 and 12 for illustrations of this). The necessity for some containment of an emotional state continues throughout life but is particularly in evidence at times of extreme stress or distress.

Sorensen opens up this concept, used with such frequency by all psychodynamic workers, to show its component parts. In doing so she reveals the complexity and richness in the concept; she illustrates, with clinical examples, how it embraces observation and the essential nature of observation to close detail before containment can take place. She links observation with Bion's ideas of Love, Hate and Knowledge. The second component of the containing process she describes as the work of clarifications and the third, emotional resonance. She emphasises that containing is an active process in which a responsive mind is performing certain tasks – focusing, discriminating and feeling, and then integrating these functions.

Chapter 8, 'Speculations on components in the infant's sense of agency: the sense of abundance and the capacity to think in parentheses', is richly illustrated by infant observation material, which allows the reader to join the debate concerning those conditions which are essential for healthy emotional and cognitive development. Anne Alvarez has made a particular contribution to psychoanalytic thinking in emphasising the interrelatedness of emotion and cognition.

In her chapter the complementary contributions of developmental researchers and psychoanalytic writers are recognised. The material illuminates the idea that any infant is dependent on a sensitive response by important caregivers to the infant's pleasurable attempts to produce a response in others. The infant's increasing pleasure in mastery over his world encourages him to learn more about it. She explores what facilitates the development of this capacity in the mother/infant relationship, a sense of 'agency' in the infant's relationship to one person and to two people. She describes the importance in the caregiver of a capacity to keep the baby in the background of the mind at moments when something or someone else is a primary preoccupation. She gives due emphasis to the equally important capacity of the caregiver to tolerate, and even value, those moments when the infant's own focus of interest maybe on someone or something other than the mother. These ideas are illuminated particularly by the beautifully detailed, but painful, observation material provided by Piera Furgiuele. This infant's difficulties are contrasted with two shorter excerpts from observations of infants who were more fortunate.

In Chapter 9, 'Psychosomatic integrations: eye and mouth in infant observation', Maria Rhode explores the interrelationship between psyche and soma, proposing an equivalence between eye and meaning on the one hand, and mouth and sensation on the other. Prompted by her experiences with an autistic patient, she explores the possibility that the over-emphasis on sensation as well as a tendency to somatisation in autism, may follow from the apprehension that real mental contact with the mind of another would be intolerable. Rhode then goes on to challenge the notion of mind developing out of bodily experiences (see Chapter 5). She uses material from three observations of different infants: the first observation provides evidence of the baby's preconception of an integrated object. It is Rhode's contention that the mother has an integrating function for the infant in being the person who thinks about what her infant might be *feeling*. The second observation illustrates the dysfunction between eye and mouth, with accompanying somatisation, when the mother was unable to acknowledge the traumatic nature of a separation. The third example illustrates a similar dysfunction, with compensatory emphasis on the physical provision of food. Here the presence of the observer, as a container for the infant's powerful emotions, is recognised as serving a healing function on behalf of the infant (the role of the observer is explored in some detail in Chapters 2, 5 and 12 in this volume).

The function by which someone outside the infant responds in a way which makes the infant aware of the effect he has produced, is linked to the idea of 'agency' explored by Alvarez and Furgiuele in Chapter 8. In her chapter, Rhode places particular emphasis on the importance of eye contact; this has considerable significance for those infants who are born blind and for their caretakers. (See Chapter 3 where one of the infants described by Jeanne Magagna is a blind baby.)

In Chapter 10, 'Interplay: sound aspects in mother–infant observation', Suzanne Maiello focuses on vocal interactions between mother and infant. She traces this back to experiences *in utero*, where the hearing capacity of the human foetus is completely developed by four months of intra-uterine life. This is linked to the notion that some form of introjection can take place before birth and that the introjected elements have, at least partly, sound qualities deriving from the child's perception of the mother's voice. (This would also include, of course, other important family members.)

Maiello draws the reader's attention to the neglect, in psychoanalytic thinking, of the importance of the acquisition at birth of a voice, which brings about the possibility of actual one-to-one vocal exchange. She discusses the importance of meeting the mother's voice again, after birth, as a realisation of what has been already internalised as a 'sound object' during pre-natal life. Vocalisation can then be understood as the expression of the internalised sound object. These ideas are supported by rich material drawn from infant observation.

The link between Chapters 9 and 10 will be apparent. Chapter 10, however, can also usefully be read in conjunction with Chapter 8. Increasing mastery in the use of the voice, enhances the infant's capacity to have an impact on mother, father, siblings and other important people in the infant's life. The emotional quality of their vocal responses will in turn provide important evidence to the infant of the degree of success in engaging their interest.

In the early days and weeks of life, the caregiver's capacity to respond with interest and warmth to the baby's first utterances will give some of the first evidence to the infant that there has been an impact on important others. Repeated experiences of this kind demonstrate to the infant that it is the infant itself who can evoke responses in others.

These are the early, loving, proto-conversational exchanges which may be observed in any ordinary family: they are characterised by warmth, by expressive facial gestures in each and by an atmosphere of pleasure. Such early 'conversations' will be initiated sometimes by the infant, sometimes by mother, but each begins to anticipate that the other will respond, and respond in a particular way. It is important that the adults and siblings in the child's world also respond intelligently, thoughtfully adapting the range of appropriate responses according to the increasing cognitive capacities shown by the baby.

Although each chapter stands very much on its own, the links between chapters are also evident. It is anticipated that the connections between the chapters will serve to clarify and amplify the often complex ideas that each author is attempting to explore.

REFERENCES

Bick, E. (1964) 'Notes on infant observation in psychoanalytic training', *International Journal of Psychoanalysis*, 45: 558–566.

Bion, W. (1962) *Learning from Experience*, London: Heinemann.

Freud, S. (1920) 'Beyond the pleasure principle', *Standard Edition* 18, London: Hogarth.

Harris, M. (1987) 'Papers on infant observation', in M. P. H. Williams, (ed.) *The Collected Papers of Martha Harris and Esther Bick*, pp. 219–239, Strath Tay, Perthshire: Clunie Press.

Klein, M. (1952) 'On observing the behaviour of young infants', in Joan Riviere (ed.) *Developments in Psychoanalysis*, London: Hogarth.

Miller, L., Rustin, M. E., Rustin, M. J. and Shuttleworth, J. (1989) *Closely Observed Infants*, London: Duckworth.

Piontelli, A. (1986) *Backward in Time: A Study in Infant Observation by the Method of Esther Bick*, Strath Tay Perthshire: Clunie Press.

Piontelli, A. (1987) 'Infant observation from before birth', *International Journal of Psycho-Analysis*, 68: 458–468.

Piontelli, A. (1992) *From Foetus to Child: An Observational and Psychoanalytic Study*, London: Routledge.

Winnicott, D. W. (1958) 'Observation of infants in a set situation', in *Collected Papers*, London: Tavistock (first published 1941).

Chapter 5

First light

Knowing the infant as an actuality and as an idea

Eric Rhode

INTRODUCTION

An observer who 'enters the field' in conducting an infant observation comes to know the infant and its caretakers directly. As it thinks about the experiences of the observer, the seminar group comes to know an experience *by hearsay*. An obvious point: and yet the two perceptions of experience involve different dimensions in intuition. While the observer undergoes the bewilderment of living through an often intense experience, the seminar group arrives at a knowledge unsupported by direct sense information and has to face different perplexities.

The observer is under pressure. The presence of a baby, or the presence of a space where a baby might be, arouses powerful feelings in a family. Being 'in the field' can inhibit the capacity, essential to observation, of being able to reverie about experience. The seminar group also has to undergo thought-inhibiting pressures, although it may find that thinking about the experiences of someone who has been in the field, without its being in the field itself, can extend the capacity to reverie.

Babies arouse envy and adoration, as well as the wish to respond to their helplessness. But the complications in feeling that arise when confronted by an actual baby are different from the complications that arise when the baby is an *idea* in a seminar group. The seminar group *can never know the baby in any direct way and has to escape from the erroneous belief that it can know the baby, in the same way as it might know a baby by way of sense knowledge.*

The idea of the baby in the seminar group has all the power that an unconscious group object can muster. A baby that is thought about, but is not directly known, is *exactly like a god who can be thought about but not known.* Aspects of its existence are liable to be strenuously denied; even though its existence as an idea is supported by the 'memories in feeling' that almost every member of the seminar group has – of siblings, offspring and, not least, of child parts of themselves.

The apportioning of a split between observer and seminar group is reminiscent of a similar apportionment in the practice of individual psychotherapy. The patient on one side of the split makes a contribution, which may be little more than a charisma of unself-conscious being, an embodiment of existence (as though the patient said 'I am what I am, nothing more, nothing less'). The therapist on the other side of the split hopes to exercise a capacity to 'dream about' the patient's contribution, in such a way that thought can translate the patient's vitality into a system of signs. It is as though embodiment, or being, had some substrate in the sign language of hallucination that has to be sought out.

ARGUMENT

Melanie Klein makes a historical or developmental distinction concerning infancy when she describes the evolution of the depressive position out of the paranoid-schizoid position as occurring during the second quarter of the first year of life (Klein 1935: 262–289). Granted: but Melanie Klein's classification may turn out to have a greater significance as describing an a-spatial and a-temporal structure from which thought derives and which logically may precede the emergence of historical and developmental considerations.

Coming to know the baby as an idea rather than as an actuality may encourage the seminar group to recall W.R. Bion's post-Kleinian understanding of intuition.

Bion realised that the journey between the two positions, which includes the crossing of a disquieting threshold between them, is a perennial state (Bion 1962). It may begin at some time in the individual's history, but the temporal metaphor of a journey is of limited value, since notions of space and time are marginal to the two positions as structural facts that exist outside space and time. Bion thought of movement between the two positions as an oscillation, persistent in states of discovery as well as in states of regression. The oscillation indicates some essential *given* in the nature of mind. The trauma of birth, if it is a trauma, is a version of the oscillation. It is *not* the starting point.

Almost in anticipation of infant observation, William Wordsworth wrote:

Our birth is but a sleep and a forgetting:
The Soul that arises with us, our life's Star,
Hath had elsewhere its setting, and cometh from afar.

(Wordsworth 1807)

If the history of the foetus were to be put into reverse as a fact of the imagination, a Platonist might argue that it seems to return to a womb-like radiant space within the womb that may owe little to biological originality. In William Golding's novel, *Darkness Visible*, a small boy walks out of a ball of fire during the London blitz, as though the core of heat had generated him.

The possibility that a preconceptive understanding of mind as originating in some light of the mind, rather than in embodiment, can arise as an idea in individual psychotherapy. In psychotic perception, body itself seems to emerge from bodily sensation. But in the rationality that I am describing, bodily experience seems to emerge from thought. It is as though experience were able to converse with the prototypes of reason.

In the beginning, there are the conjoined good objects, defined by Donald Meltzer (in discussion) as objects of radiance. The objects impel a desire for notation. Descartes wrote to a colleague: 'I believe that the soul is always thinking for the same reason as I believe that light is always shining, even though there are not always eyes looking at it' (Descartes 1642). An emotional *turbulence* arises: Bion's oscillation between the two positions. Out of turbulence may stem an experience and knowledge of body.

The observer in the field and the seminar group will begin by engaging with the actuality in which the newborn lives. Obviously it is important to strengthen the down-to-earth aspects of the observer's relationship to the field and to endorse the fact that cogency of insight depends on an element of common sense in perception. But it is important, too, that the seminar group should be invited to share the experience of another type of perception – that of being agents for the 'eyes of the mind', for reason itself, by being attentive to intuitions of a preconceptive kind, concerning structures in thought that are like forms in music.

Thinking of this kind is characteristic of myth, and I shall trace its influence on an observation brought to a certain seminar group.

THE FISH MOBILE

The observer met the family before the birth of Anna and brought the observation to the group. I shall allude to this observation in passing. She made an observation after the birth which she did not present to the group, and then an observation which she did present.

> Anna is twelve days old. Joseph lets me in [Joseph is aged eleven and is Anna's one sibling]. Anna's mother is sitting over Anna, who is feeding quietly at the right breast. Mother explains that Anna started crying badly half-way home from school – they had been collecting Joseph – and that she rushed her back under her coat with Joseph pushing the pram home.
>
> Joseph goes to fetch the sweets that I brought for him last week, and offers me one, then offers the bag to his mother who asks him to unwrap one and to pop it in her mouth.
>
> Joseph points out the fish mobile that he has made. I now realise that

he had been making the fish mobile during my first visit, before Anna
had been born.

During the first visit, Joseph had been busy working with pen and paper
and scissors, and the observer had had no clue as to what he had been
making; and this sense of mystery had seemed to reflect the sense of an
event that was about to happen (the birth of Anna).

> During the feed Anna strains and seems to have a bowel motion. Mum
> says that the trouble now is that she has got herself all upset and is
> now feeding and probably windy. But in fact she probably is hungry as
> she didn't have much before she went out, and she's gone an hour and
> a half. Mum says that Anna has to fit into a routine unlike Joseph did.

Anna comes off the right breast in some distress. The observer takes note
that Anna 'strains' and 'seems to have a bowel motion' under the influence
of her mother's anxiety; or at least her mother is anxious, and Anna has
had a bowel motion. Mother has had to race to school with Anna to
collect Anna's elder brother Joseph and now has hoped to feed her to make
her less anxious. While mother feeds Anna, Joseph pops a consolatory
sweet into his mother's mouth.

In a remark of some resonance, Anna's mother says that Anna has a
way of coming off the breast when upset that suggests she may have
forgotten it, or does not know where it is, or has rejected it. Her response
to the 'upset' is to suppose that Anna, as the second child, has not as yet
had time to realise that she 'has to fit into a routine.' On first phoning the
observer, she had apologised for her baby because, she said, 'this was a
second baby'. The observer told the seminar group, 'I may have com-
pounded that feeling of second best by saying honestly that I didn't have
a choice.' Mother was glad to take her on (the observer was to learn)
because of the family's good experience with a first observer, a speech
therapist who had helped them all by her presence and whose capacity
for observation may have fostered Joseph's precocity in speech. 'I
wondered what gifts they expected from me', the second observer thought
ruefully.

Sue Reid (in discussion) has suggested that the notion of 'second best'
works against any understanding of the obvious fact that every baby is
unique. In this context, being second best probably means being a girl.
(We never learn why Anna's mother has had all the time in the world for
Joseph but has so little time for Anna.)

The reiteration of secondness invites comparison with some idealised
conception of the foetus's relationship to the umbilical cord, in which
functions of feeding and evacuation are not necessarily separated or liable
to interruption.

Joseph translucently reflects the family's phantasies and feelings. On first seeing him, the observer had noted that he looked like his father; but her observation brought out the extent to which Joseph seemed to be immersed in his mother's pregnancy. Much of the hostility that Joseph might reasonably have felt at the birth of the new baby was avoided by his immersion; he might have been in a *couvade*, or phantom pregnancy state, as his mother realises. She says that Joseph is 'a bit full' of himself; he 'has really got into the pregnancy'. She adds: 'He has read all the books on pregnancy'.

It is as though Joseph had become confused with an *idea* of the foetus. His state of confusion has only begun to be shaken a little by his first meetings with an actual sister. He cannot really see her, nor can his mother, because they are lost in an idea which both of them believe can have only one embodiment – as a boy (and a specific boy at that: Joseph) rather than as a girl (Anna).

Joseph possibly speaks for his mother's intuitions, most noticeably so when the observer, on first meeting the family before Anna's birth, had observed his making of the fish mobile, without understanding what he was about. Later in this same first observation, Joseph's mother had talked about puzzling over some ultrasound photographs of Anna *in utero*, which she thought of disparagingly as being like 'a toddler's picture, in which people have the head pointed out and then say "Oh yes, how very nice".' Mother's looking into the womb, by way of the ultrasound, echoes Joseph's need to construct an imaginary or dreamlike image of the womb, the fish mobile made as a gift for a baby that is to be and yet is unknown, like a preconception that awaits realisation, or a thought in the mind of the seminar group.

By the fact that it does not have the experiential knowledge of the observer, the seminar group is in a position to see with 'the eyes of the mind' the significance of the fish mobile as an actual event that has a strong dream component to it. As a dream representation, the fish mobile depicts poetically, as depressive threshold symbols tend to do, the fundamental mystery or ambivalence of life and death as presences in the mind.

We can now see the significance of the relationship of doubling to the theme of otherness. The eyes of actual perception are to 'the eyes of the mind' as the actual infant is to the imaginary twin in the breast, who carries an other-worldly capacity to tolerate the existence of some essential mystery in life and death.

Joseph speaks for the family, and in particular for his mother, through his making of the gift, as though for a baby in a manger.

The fish mobile should symbolise the realisation of an inner world depressive space, in which the idea of the *otherness* of the imaginary twin can be tolerated. But in fact, Joseph's gift is not used in the service of Anna; it is used as a defence against realising a jealousy that is on the verge of being activated by her unique claims on life. Although this realisation cannot be tolerated, its meaning is evident as an unconsciously shared family phantasy, at the time when Anna reaches the second breast.

Anna comes off the first breast in some distress, and her mother says that she is not sure whether Anna 'forgets' the breast, or somehow loses it, or just doesn't want it. (In the same way as mother and Joseph want to 'forget' the unique particularity of the second baby.) At this moment, Anna's mother and Joseph are more distanced than Anna is from an idea of integrating goodness. Caught up in a phantasy about the meaning of Anna's bowel motion, they share states of mind that are characterised by an absence of moderation.

> Anna's mother says, 'It's alright Anna, it's alright' and holds her close. Anna's mother is trying to wind her and takes her upstairs for a nappy change. On the way upstairs she turns up the thermostat, saying that her husband is worried about overheating, and 65 degrees is now recommended because of cot death.

On the changing mat Anna looks at the window and 'moves rhythmically and alternately' and 'makes little noises in her throat'. She now carries the mystery of otherness. What do her movements mean, if anything? Is she trying to hold onto an internal good that she has projected on to the world outside her? But mother and Joseph are unable to see her at this moment. Rather, Joseph feigns perturbation at the 'orange-coloured poo'; and mother and he enter into a crescendo of anxiety concerning the theme of being pushed out, or denied rights. Since Anna's birth, says Joseph, he has had to use his parents' toilet, though why he has had to do so is not clear; and Anna's mother talks about a sewer failure, and about a neighbour whose toilet had been blocked. Things are getting out of hand and, as though to get a grip on herself, Anna's mother says that she uses liners and terry-towel nappies which date from Joseph's time.

When Anna begins to scream, Joseph seems to become genuinely persecuted. He puts his hands over his ears, rushes away and lies on his parents' bed with a pillow over either ear. It is as though the screaming and defecating were equated with the act of Anna's conception, perhaps in this very bed. Feeding and hearing in the actual world entails being able to take in a sibling's screams: the insistence of new life to be acknowledged.

In the conjectures of the seminar group, the thought of Joseph with pillows over his ears is as dreamlike as the image of the fish mobile. Imagination might see the image of Joseph with his ears covered as though through an *enfilade* of rooms, or as existing within the incoherent spaces that typify the labile space–time intuitions of the depressive threshold.

In certain contexts, the 'eyes of the mind' have the magnifying powers of a telescope or microscope. I take this counter-transference response to contain an understanding about the changes in psychic space that the activity of birth stirs up in the phantasies of a family involved in the experience of an actual birth.

In the observation group, as it thinks about the material, psychic meaning can manifest itself as though alternating through either a microscope or telescope. It is as though this unsecured type of perception (oral in origin, I suspect) were a prerequisite for being able to 'see' by way of the 'eye of the mind'. Intuitions of this kind oscillate between microcosmic and macrocosmic conceptions of understanding.

A new baby invites the thought that *it*, a minute particular, *is* the whole world: it invites thinking that is close to the concrete equation thinking that Hanna Segal has described as psychopathological (Segal 1957), but that can be on occasion (as here) used in the service of development. On this point, microcosm *is* macrocosm, as the earliest cosmologists used to believe.

Many families find themselves on the threshold as they undergo the creative turbulence of meeting up with the otherness of a new life – and extraordinary conceptions of space and time can be evidence of the depressive threshold. The observer, as opposed to the seminar leader, is seldom in the position to acknowledge this sort of response; 'having an actual experience', and being bombarded by it, can inhibit the capacity to receive this type of insight. The seminar group acknowledges the truth in actuality in the description of a circumstance, while at the same time 'seeing' quite different lines of thought for exploration.

Mother now takes a hold on the situation: she sends off Joseph to finish his homework and brings Anna to the second breast, from which Anna feeds keenly.

Anna cries a little at the end of her feed, and her mother helps to settle her by putting on a tape recording of the kind of sounds that a foetus might hear in the womb. Arguably, Anna's mother is trying to fob off Anna once more. To that extent, she is mis-using her intuition. But perhaps she lacks confidence in the power of the breast to settle little girls as well as little boys.

> Anna is quiet – half awake and half asleep – and then her face creases up and she cries quite suddenly. Her mother puts on a tape of womb noises, and Anna seems to relax very quickly and to fall asleep, hanging over her mother's arms. Her mother says that the tape seems to work and that classical music has the same effect.

This is to think of classical music as a type of sedation, used to control the mind rather than to open it to the truth. Ideas that genuinely belong to the inner world are powerful forms of good, but they can be abused. For instance: cultures haunted by ideas at the expense of being attuned to actualities tend to be oppressive of individuality, even though the ideas are valuable in themselves.

And yet Anna's mother does have an intuition so stimulating that it led to the writing of this paper. Linking classical music to womb sounds indicates an understanding of a way in which the earliest self may delight in its good objects as a type of *proportionality*. A passion for music or mathematics may grow out of such a delight.

As the tape of womb sounds continues, Anna's mother mentions bringing Anna home a few days before – in a way that anticipates, but in a more happy key, the anxious homecoming of today. She and her husband had enjoyed giving Anna a bath, and Anna had enjoyed the bath too. It was as though, through womb sounds and music and water, and the experience of Anna entering sleep drowsily, mother and the observer had been allowed a glimpse of the unknowable core to the dream element. Hopefully the seminar group is sensitive to this unknowable core.

CONCLUSION

The mysterious and radiant environment of the newborn creates a formidable field for the observer to travel into.

Imaginatively identified with the foetus, the seminar group may see the observer as the foetus's own later infant self, hesitantly contemplating a new world and looking to find its anchorage in its foetal past. The intrepidity of the observer may put the seminar group in mind of early navigators sailing through uncharted waters.

In relation to the actions of other members of the family, the newborn (as when it looks at the light from a window or turns its head) has a metaphysical 'depth' that is mysterious; it seems to be looking for something, and to embody something, which the actual world can only reflect uncertainly.

I conjecture that what it is looking for is something that comes from a world of non-naturalistic proto-spatial and proto-temporal intuitions that is relatable only secondarily to foetal intuition.

The seminar group, and possibly the observer, may sense how close the infant is to the radiance of the good objects. The observer, blitzed by sensation and erroneous advice from 'bad' figures from within, is under pressure to think in terms of a delusional certainty that derives from a misunderstanding of empiricism. The seminar group, on the other hand, may feel an appeal that is related to the evolution of sign systems that occur within the non-successive and often 'alien' spatial conceptions of dream thought.

Freud wrote in *Moses and Monotheism* of an 'intellectuality' drained of 'sensory perception' that is required to contemplate a God who has 'neither a name nor a countenance' (Freud 1939: 113). 'Intellectuality' is a native endowment, a structure in reasoning which the foetus can intuit, one of the earliest forms by which good objects articulate meaning to the mind.

The seminar group has some responsibility to strengthen the down-to-earth, commonsense inclinations of the observer, while at the same time bearing witness to the fact that thought actually exists and that mind is structured in an 'intellectuality' that contemplates an articulation 'without a name or a countenance'. An experience of the actual in itself, without the dream element (if this can be imagined), would be unable to convey the experience of mind being able to come to suffer the nature of its own unknowability.

REFERENCES

Bion, W. R. (1962) *Learning from Experience*, London: Heinemann.

Descartes, R. (1642) 'Letter to Gibieuf', 19 January 1642, in A. Kenny (ed.) *Descartes' Philosophical Letters*, Oxford Clarendon Press.

Freud, S. (1939) *Moses and Monotheism, Standard Edition* 23, London: The Hogarth Press.

Golding, W. (1979) *Darkness Visible*, London: Faber and Faber.

Kenny, A. (ed.) (1970) *Descartes' Philosophical Letters*, Oxford: Clarendon Press.

Klein, M. (1935) 'A contribution to the psychogenesis of manic-depressive states', in *The Writings of Melanie Klein*, Volume 1, edited by R. Money-Kyrle, in collaboration with B. Joseph, E. O'Shaughnessy and H. Segal, London: Hogarth Press (1975).

Segal, H. (1957) 'Notes on symbol formation', *International Journal of Psycho-Analysis*, 38: 391–397.

Wordsworth, W. (1807) 'Ode: Intimations of Immortality from Recollections of Early Childhood', in *Wordsworth: Poetry and Prose*, selected by W. M. Merchant, London: Rupert Hart-Davies (1955).

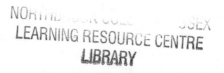

Chapter 6

Moments of discovery, times of learning

Alex Dubinsky and Olga Bazhenova

INTRODUCTION

This chapter is concerned with the vicissitudes of the interest that mother
and infant take in the manifestations of each other's mind. Starting with
the attention given to the eyes and the voice, we will consider how this
interest plays an important role in the early months as it helps the
emotional relationship between mother and child both to be sustained and
to develop.

We will base this discussion on material from the infant observation
seminar at the Faculty of Psychology of the State University of Moscow.
The observation of baby Sasha was made by Ludmila Baz. The observation
of the second baby, Masha, was made by Tat'yana Petriky. Both observers
kindly allowed us to make use of their notes.

PARASITIC AND COMMENSAL DEVELOPMENT

Love, and an awareness that the baby has a mind, are not sufficient for
the establishment of a commensal relationship between mother and child.
(Bion defined as commensal a relationship conducive to growth for both
protagonists and for the relation (Bion 1970: 95).) Interest in the manifestations of each other's mind is required for this purpose.

This will be illustrated by a difficult period in the relationship between
baby Sasha and his perceptive, affectionate but depressed mother, Anna.
She is in her early twenties and lives with her two parents. Her husband
lives separately because the apartment is very small. Sasha is their first
baby. For the first month he had been crying most of the time and the
family asked the observer to postpone her visit.

The baby was therefore five weeks old by the time of the first observation. His name had only just been chosen. Until now he had simply
been called 'the little one'. Anna was sitting in an armchair, huddling
together with the sleeping baby under a blanket, as she felt frozen after a
walk. This was to be the first indication that she was identifying with a hurt
child. She started by talking to the observer about the baby's physical

problems: there was concern about the joints in his feet and the possible need for a plaster cast. The frenulum on his tongue was also too short and caused him to swallow air when he sucked. Sasha was asleep, lying against his mother's chest and belly with his head against her cheek. Anna described his sleeping in the open air as his 'switching off'. As the baby became agitated, she caressed his hand and his forehead. The baby cried without waking up.

> Affectionately Mummy says to him 'Little one, what is it?' She holds him in a way which is more comfortable for him, lifts him up and tells me that's how it is when they have wind and then to him again: 'Does it hurt you? Does it hurt?' Anna's attention appears to help him. For a few minutes the baby seems asleep, but now the globes of his eyes are moving under the eyelids, his mouth opens up and his lips move as if he is sucking. Anna says affectionately: 'He is dreaming.' She is indeed quite observant and perceptive. Sasha wakes up a minute or two later, it seems to me that he is opening his eyes – at first, little slits, then his eyes disappear, and then at last they are open, with his gaze fixed in the direction of the window. His mother says, laughing: 'We call this the contemplation of the world.' The baby is lying with his gaze gradually turning to my side, then he looks at the ceiling and then again at the window. He is sucking his fist.

Sasha has been comforting himself in his sleep, perhaps by dreaming of the breast. When he wakes up we see that he doesn't search for his mother's face or fasten on the observer but instead holds himself to the light while still trying to re-create the experience of feeding at the breast by sucking his fist.

Anna told the observer of his interest in the red lamp-shade on the table where she changes him, and also of the toy she shows him 'when he is in a good mood'. Sasha cried and she gave him the dummy, asking him 'Little one, will this distract you?' She explained to the observer that according to Dr Spock, babies suck their fists when they have tummy pain. The baby fell asleep.

Anna gave the baby to his grandmother, who went with him to another room. When mother and the observer joined them, Grandmother told them that the baby was very hot; that he must have become too hot when he was with his mother under the woollen blanket. Anna began to worry and spent a long time placing a thermometer under the baby's tiny hand. As he cried, Grandmother told him something tenderly and with expression (that he was a good boy, etc.). He listened and looked in her face. When he was found to have a temperature of 37.1°C everybody worried (although it is a normal temperature), but Grandmother was reassuring: he had been too hot, and she suggested that he be given something to drink, which Mother did.

Later Mother changes his nappy. All that time he is lying with his head turned to the left – there are his beloved lamp and his toy. Mother lifts his toy. He turns his head and follows it. As he finds himself on his right side, he tries to turn his head to the left as far as he can: there stands his favourite lamp. Mother laughs.

We see that Sasha is focusing his attention on material objects, not on his mother's face, and that she is not calling his attention to herself.

The baby soon falls asleep in his bed, then cries, wakes up and wants to be fed. Grandmother takes him to the bathroom. Sasha is up in the air, resting with his tummy on the palm of his grandmother's hand, arms and legs hanging down, but he is holding up his head. Finding himself suddenly in such an unexpected situation he opens his eyes wide, his gaze is moving in various directions. His little face looks surprised, his mouth is open, his lower lip is sticking out. And then his gaze stops on my face, and there are a few seconds of tense examination: there are wrinkles on his forehead and frowning folds between his eyebrows. And suddenly, oh miracle! he directs a broad smile at me. I am ecstatic. However, he has already heard the sound of water running and with a contented look on his face he is letting himself be washed . . .

Exchanges such as this one helped us to recognise the nature of the difficulties in the relationship between Mother and Sasha. Ordinarily, these exchanges are privileged moments in the life of a mother and her baby. They are stepping-stones on the path of development as they support a certain kind of reciprocal relationship. It is characterised by a spirit of enquiry and a shared sense of wonder and delight at having access to the other's mind.

Together with a sensitive understanding of the baby by his mother there needs to be a mutual curiosity. It would seem that it is the inherent creativity of the mind which invites the other to enquire into its new manifestations. From the mother's and the baby's facial expressions as representations of their emotional state, to the tone, modulation, accentuation and rhythm of the voice, to simple play, to words . . . the series is actually infinite and invites an ever-extending enquiry, provided Love and Hate are attended to (Bion regarded loving, hating and knowing 'as intrinsic to the link between [people] considered to be in relationship with each other' (Bion 1962:42)). For Vygotsky, giving meaning to the elements in this series is actually the basis of psychic development. (Vygotsky 1960: 1984).

Neither Mother nor Sasha was seeking a commensal relation based on such a mutual desire to know the other. Although the baby enjoyed the moments of mutual attention with the observer and with his grandmother, he was not attempting to prolong them. Neither was he trying to catch the attention of Mother's eyes. We need here to acknowledge that there are significant aspects of the relation between them about which we have no information: for instance, what emotion was Mother conveying to the baby when he was crying inconsolably during the first weeks? Why was it that only his beloved grandfather could comfort him?

> Let us now return to the observation, when somewhat later Mother gets ready to feed the baby. There is a pillow on the bed and next to it a nappy where the baby is placed with his face slightly turned to the right, towards the cushion. Mother lies next to him on her left side. He wriggles discontentedly but quietens down once he finds the breast and sucks avidly. His eyes are closed, his hands are tightened into a fist, close to his cheeks, with their backs facing each other. Sasha is making loud noises. Mother explains that he is swallowing some air. He sucks energetically for ten minutes, then dozes off. Mother smiles at her son and calls him 'a suckling piglet'. She moves the nipple and he suddenly remembers to make a few sucking movements. All this time, Mother has been holding either one or the other of his hands, removing a speck of dust, caressing his little forehead.

The feeding position suggests something more limited than a full embrace. Mother appears to think that the breast is all that she can offer and that it is all that interests the baby, this 'piglet' she loves tenderly. In fact, Sasha seems to concentrate entirely on the feeding. But let us return again to the observation.

> Mother says that she would like Sasha to talk early, but that her friend has a little boy who is two years and two months old and only has a few words. Mother adds: 'My mum says that I talk too little to him and that, with me, he will learn to speak late, but somehow I can't manage to do it.'

Mother feels affectionate towards Sasha but experiences their relationship as restricted (if only he could talk . . . if only she could not be disappointed like her friend whose child only says a few words . . .). She does not think that Sasha has something to offer to her mind now. When Anna says that she is unable to talk to him she is linking, in her conscious associations, this state of affairs to her own limitations. The way she puts it is informative: 'My mum says . . .'. She speaks like a little girl who has been told off by a mother possessed of every competence.

Anna is also drawing attention to an actual limitation in her talking to the baby. It is not that she doesn't talk to him but that she does not appear to address him directly except about pain and comfort. She was not trying to engage him when she called him a 'suckling piglet' or when later that afternoon she told him: 'Little one, did you understand yourself what you want?' as the sleeping baby seemed ready to cry but contented himself with a few groans. It is speech which is not expected to initiate a communication with the baby but is instead intended to be heard by herself, or the observer. Dr Lynne Murray, who has researched extensively into the relationship between depressed mothers and their babies, recently gave a lecture with an evocative title starting with the words: 'Speech without communication'. Progressively, a sense of Anna's psychological depletion is emerging.

In the next observation, Sasha was six weeks old. Anna told the observer that he now slept for long periods in the day, for up to seven or eight hours. She was finding this difficult as she did not know whether to wake him up. Sasha was sleeping in his pram, and Anna said that he was not deeply asleep, and that he would wake up soon.

> But little Sasha is not waking up: at times his eyeballs move under the closed eyelids, at times they stop and it seems that he is opening his eyes – two slits appear. After some time his little mouth opens, his upper lip protrudes and his chin starts to move – as if he were making sucking movements. After a few such movements comes a halt, a few deep noisy sighs, and the little boy again seems to suck. There is quiet for some time but then he lets out a strange cry (his mother calls it the 'cry of the Red Indians') and the pram moves as the little boy lifts his legs and pulls them to his tummy. His head turns to the left, then back; he wrinkles his face and shouts a few times. We think that he has woken up and that he shouts out of hunger ('Enough, it is time') but suddenly the baby takes his previous position and quietens down. In fact his eyes do not open . . . . This went on for another twenty minutes. Mother and the observer then left the room.

Sasha was withdrawing into sleep and seemed to be dreaming of feeding at the breast. When he was awake, the moments of emotional intensity with his mother were focused on the feeding itself. He was turning away from a relationship with her which would go beyond the feeding, to involve looking and listening. When later that afternoon Anna fed him, Sasha sucked avidly at the breast with his hands closed in a fist. She was probably expressing her sense that he was only relating to part of her when she told him: 'My pump works well, eh, Sasha?'

After the feed, Anna held the baby upright with his back against her chest. After he burped, Mother and observer noticed that he was fixing something with concentration but they couldn't tell what it was. The observer's face came close to the baby's face.

> His gaze moves and meets mine . . . he studies me attentively, opening his little mouth, he creases his forehead, he turns himself to the right with a smile, then again turning back he looks at me, again smiles and turns away; he does this a few times. Mother laughs: 'You are like a

pretty girl.' She then offers him toys but he does not look at them until she shakes his favourite rattle. He turns his gaze on her and then gives out some sort of a sound and lets his head down: Mother thinks this is a sign that he is tired.

This moment of the observation leaves one with a poignant sense of an encounter that does not take place. It also seems that for Sasha the emotional link is painful.

In her conversation with the observer that afternoon, Anna recounted that in the past she had laughed when she had read that mothers got depressed after the baby's birth but now she could see it was true. External factors had made a significant contribution to this internal situation. There was worry about the baby having suffered physical damage before he was born. The baby's continuous crying in the first week was painful to hear. The family later suggested that it might have been colic. Anna and her husband had to live separated and she must have missed his support. Anna lived on the fourth floor and there was no lift: she only very rarely went out of the very small apartment during the first two months. The observation also showed that her own mother was projecting inadequacy into Anna and was subtly disparaging of her. Anna was still very young, and she had been quite hurt when she did not get a university place before she decided to work as a nurse. She complained to the observer, wondering when she would open a book again now that she had a baby.

Anna talked of how some mothers do not like it when their own mother gave them advice: with her it was the opposite, she didn't know what she would have done without her Mum. She always reassured her. Anna went on: 'Not long ago we cut into his finger when we were doing his nails. For two days I was afraid he would get septicaemia'.

It appears that in Anna's internal world babies were constantly exposed to damage and in need of preventive or reparative care. An all-competent super-ego seemed to point to the dreadful consequences of her imagined incompetence. Doctors' concerns about the baby only served to confirm Anna's anxieties. Her identification with a baby, both hurt and helpless, further contributed to her sense of inadequacy. Also, like many mothers, she had lost the support to her identity as an adult which a professional occupation provides.

The observations also suggest that she felt she lacked the resources to evoke the child's interest. At that time there did not seem to be any figures in her internal world to encourage and inspire her. It is probably because she projected her sense of depletion that she perceived the baby as having little to offer her. This sense of depletion also brought a fear of change which she expressed when she said: 'Earlier I kept talking of how one would like everything to remain stable so that one would know what he would come up with. Now I understand that this is not possible.'

Both Anna and Sasha were turning away from new shared experience. This was hindering the development of the relationship, despite the mutual affection. While the baby was concentrating on the pleasures of feeding, Anna was expressing her love and assuaging her depressive anxieties through taking care of him physically. These physical interactions were becoming their main shared activity.

The mobilisation of the means to avoid new experience and thus discovery, renders the relationship between mother and child detrimental to the growth of the two protagonists and of the relationship. It becomes what Bion called a parasitic relationship (Bion 1970: 95). Learning from experience, whether through discovering new aspects of the other, or through discovering new aspects of their own personality, is curtailed for both mother and child. Moreover, this turning away means that neither is offering the other the much-needed encouragement to develop the relationship.

DISCOVERING THE MANIFESTATIONS OF THE OTHER'S MIND

We will now turn to the observation of Masha. Her mother is in her early twenties and lives with her husband and her parents. From early on Masha showed a spirit of enquiry and a passionate responsiveness. When the observer first saw her she was five weeks old, like Sasha.

She is lying on her back on a nappy spread on the sofa. She is gently moving her legs and her arms, and looks with curiosity at times at the ceiling, at times at her mother, at times to the side. Mother is sitting next to the child while watching television and knitting. After some time Mother turns to the baby. She says tenderly, looking into her eyes: 'agoo, agoo' and tries to put the dummy in her mouth. When Mother talks to the little girl she looks in her mother's eyes, but as soon as Mother tries to put the dummy in her mouth, the baby briskly turns her head away and purses her lower lip so that Mother does not succeed in her attempt. Mother starts to stroke the little girl's tummy with her left hand and speaks tenderly to the child. Masha looks at her mother, smiles broadly, and Mother then puts the dummy in the child's mouth with her right hand. The little girl starts to suck. Mother sits next to Masha looking attentively at her, and then gets up and goes out of the room. The little girl stays on her back, looking at features around her. She lifts her head and tries to see the tapestry hung on the wall behind her, then she looks up to the left, after which she tries to bend her back as much as she could, helping herself with her legs and arms, in order to see the bright pattern on the cushion at the end of the sofa. She looks with concentration at some feature for a definite period of time, then looks at something else and looks at it also for some time while sucking quietly at her dummy, stopping from time to time when she makes big efforts to move her head.

In this first observation, Masha was expectantly looking out for objects around her. She was holding on to them with her eyes in the way described by Mrs Bick (Bick 1986: 297) but at the same time found them interesting and studied them one after the other. However, her mother's eyes and talk were far more important to her than inanimate objects. Even though Mummy's intention was to give her the dummy and leave the room, Masha responded to her affectionate voice and touch with a broad smile. When she was left on her own she was capable of turning again to the things around her. Masha was also using her sense of hearing by itself despite the sound of the television in the background, and she would stay still when she could hear her mother's and her grandmother's voices coming from the kitchen.

In the next observation, Masha, then two months old, kept demanding from her mother the sort of attention which would provide her with a focus, something onto which she could then hold. But, as we will see, her curiosity was ready to seize upon the new noise that her mother made.

Mother starts to talk with Masha: 'But what is the matter with you? Agoo, agoo.' She then clicks her tongue to distract her daughter. When her mother takes her in her arms, the little girl quietens down. She looks with concentration at her mother, sucking rhythmically at her dummy while moving continuously the fingers of her little hands, which she keeps pressed against her chest. When mother starts to click her tongue, the little girl stays still and her eyes open wide.

Mother was obviously affectionate and concerned but she seemed often to want to move away from Masha. She was thinking about the little girl from the outside as she didn't endow her with an inner life of thoughts and feelings but only with habits. While at this point in the observation the baby was showing herself to be uncomfortable and to want attention, mother could only comment: 'She likes that one takes her in one's arms, she likes that one talks to her.'

The family soon told the observer that Masha was crying a lot. The observer felt concerned for Mother, who had slowed down in her movements and gave the impression that she was depressed. She also felt puzzled as Mother's talk to the baby was very rare and mostly limited to stereotyped baby talk.

Mother seemed to engage the child mainly to reassure herself that the baby was well. The attention that she could give to the baby seemed to be constrained by two forms of persecutory feelings. On the one hand, she appeared to be pursued by internalised figures who 'knew'. This reflected the external reality as her own mother would actually assert that she knew better. A nurse herself, Mother also seemed to be constricted by some form of internalised medical advice as she would breast-feed the child by the clock. On the other hand she also seemed unable to contain her own anxieties about the baby's well-being and she became persecuted. She could not tolerate the child's crying and demanding attention from her and on one upsetting occasion she covered the baby's eyes with a nappy as she wanted her to sleep. She kept watching thrillers on the permanently switched on television set as if she needed to reassure herself that some form of life was still going on. Emotional blindness to the mental life of the baby was a way of avoiding contact with the child's painful experiences.

In the case of Sasha, the first baby described, the problem was different. His mother could imagine a mental life for him but she could not relate to it, apparently because she perceived him as uninterestingly identical to the damaged baby self she carried inside, in phantasy. As she identified with him, she confused his mental life with her own intellectual life, which she saw as thwarted.

As for Masha, she battled on bravely. She pursued with constancy and enthusiasm her quest to discover the world through her interest in her mother. The excerpt of an observation which follows shows how she made use of times when her mother became more available. She was then three months and ten days old.

> The little girl is lying on the sofa on her back in her usual position. On each side of her is a bright rubber toy and Masha looks attentively at them in turn. Mother is sitting next to her, knitting and watching television. She seems not to have quite woken up. She hasn't done her hair and at times she yawns. There is an atmosphere of comfort and indolence in the room. Mother puts aside her knitting and with a quiet smile says in her pleasant and rather muffled voice: 'And why don't you talk, Masha, speak.' As soon as the little girl hears her mother's voice she turns her head towards her and, while looking attentively in her mother's eyes, she smiles broadly. She is trying to make sounds like 'Ah-ah, eh-eh', but she can't produce them easily as her dummy is in the way. Mother takes out the dummy, saying: 'We'll take it away, why do we need it?' The little girl continues to look attentively in her mother's eyes and starts to vocalise, drawing out the sound and changing the pitch: 'A-a-a-a.'

For a while mother and child are responding to each other in a continued dialogue. The baby's vocalisations have their place next to the looking into Mother's eyes and the broad smile. The verbal component of the relationship is developing and is taking a large part in establishing and sustaining the emotional link. For instance, when she is drawing out her vocalisations, Masha is again engaging her mother's attention while expressing and communicating her sense of its continuity.

The verbal link had evolved from Masha's initial interest in her mother's voice. She was now internalising a talking mother she could 'talk to'. This will become apparent in the next extract from the observation, when Masha transfers her interest to the toys with a new variety in her vocalisations.

When the baby was holding on to her mother's eyes while she was vocalising, she was not clinging but holding on to her good object. Together with this object, Masha was internalising a relationship which was found to be good, and interesting, and sustainable. Love and the desire to know are here intertwined in their promotion of development. However, as we will now see, Mother was still inclined to limit the relationship to establishing that the child was 'functioning' well.

> Mother looks approvingly at the little girl, saying: 'This is how we talk', and she wipes a few drops of saliva from around the child's mouth. She then turns back to the television and to her knitting. The little girl switches her attention to her toys. Looking at the big fish she says: 'Ghi-ghi, hhh, bah'. She starts to move her lips without making a sound, sometimes extending them, sometimes pursing her lower lip, and then she starts to produce bubbles of saliva and gurgling noises. She is very enthusiastic about this occupation.

Talking to the fish represented for Masha keeping up her relationship with a good mother who talked to her. These are the beginnings of symbolisation. The silent moving of the lips and the saliva bubbles suggest that the baby then turned to an exploration of the practical mechanics of communication. But the bubbles, like the sounds she had first addressed to the fish, seem also to be a projection and symbolisation of the good internalised experience.

> Mother turns to her daughter and says: 'But why don't you talk, speak?' At the same time she presses repeatedly on the fish which unexpectedly produces a loud and piercing noise. The little girl livens up, her eyes light up, with all her body she tries to turn towards the fish and she begins to vocalise energetically. Masha seems to believe she had met a talking fish! Mother laughs and presses on the other toy a few times. It makes a different sound to which the little girl also responds. Mother and daughter begin to play. Mother presses a few times on the toy, then waits for her daughter's reply, and then passes on the other toy. This is repeated a few times.

Mother and child were discovering that they could play together. Mother, however, was not able to sustain the emotional link.

After this, Mother watches television again. The little girl turns away from Mother, she is lying on her back, moving her hands and feet gently. All of a sudden, her gaze falls on the fingers of her hand which are closing and opening. She becomes interested in this, her eyes widen, the movement of the other extremities slows down. For some time the little girl looks attentively at her fingers. While she is doing this, she is at times lifting her hand a little, at times letting it come down close to the sofa. The little girl is watching the movements of her hand as if she is observing the movements of a foreign object moving independently of her will. Eventually, as she becomes bored, she stops following the trajectory of her hand.

Masha appeared to have felt dropped from her mother's attention. Nevertheless, she was able to turn to her own resources. It is not that she was just holding on to the movement of her fingers and hand. She was curious about them. She was distributing to other objects her passionate interest for the mother she had internalised.

When her hand is lifted up a little the next time, her eyes continue to fix in the same direction and meet the rubber toy, which has been previously hidden by her hand. When she sees the toy the little girl shows surprise. At this moment her hand, with the fingers moving, comes down and covers the object. The expression on Masha's face shows even more surprise. Her little hand goes up again and she sees the toy again. This is repeated a few times and it seems that Masha is consciously trying to lift up her hand again to see the toy after she has become tired and has let her hand drop back on the sofa.

CONCLUSION

These observations remind us that the very stuff, the very tissue of an emotional relationship is made not only of love and hate, but also of a passionate interest in the manifestations of the other's mind.

When it can be deployed, the infant's commitment to discovery is at first turned primarily towards his mother's eyes which fix their attention on the baby's eyes, and towards her loving voice which produces the most interesting combinations of sounds. When the mother is able to relate emotionally to her baby, she delights in the infant's freshly revealed mental abilities, which also reassure her that the baby is really alive and well. This pleasure, which is shared with the baby, is an encouragement to engage the child's attention again, while the reassurance the mother receives through these exchanges removes some of the obstacles that exaggerated depressive or persecutory anxiety might place between her and the baby. (Depressive anxiety corresponds to concern for the child's well-being and fears for the child's survival. In the case of persecutory anxiety the mother feels that she is not doing enough for the baby in the eyes of internal or external figures, or that the infant's demands are preventing her attending to her own needs.)

The importance given, on either part, to these manifestations of the other's mind contributes to the sustaining of the relationship. Mothers become interested in the emerging complexity of their baby's mental development, babies savour their increasing capacity to engage their mother's attention. Sustaining the relationship makes learning possible, both in the sense of learning about each other and in terms of internalising the good experience.

It is interesting to note that it was shown by Stroganova, a researcher at the Institute for Brain Research in Moscow, that the pleasure an infant experiences when making use of his or her knowledge is reflected by the same pattern of brainwave activity in the EEG as the one observed when the infant is kissed by his mother (Nikitina *et al.* 1987). One might think of this result as a pointer reminding us that understanding is an emotional experience, coloured by passion, as in Bion's description (Bion 1962: 42).

One could possibly limit in a behaviouristic manner the account of a baby's emotional relationship with the mother to the response to the manifestations of her mind. It seems quite legitimate however to assume that the baby has a sense that there is 'something' which is part of the mother and which presents the baby with these manifestations. This 'something' is what we, as adults, call the mind. We are then entitled to say that the baby has the experience of the mother's mind. Such a formulation does not presuppose that the baby has abstracted a concept of mind.

Explicit in psychoanalytic object relationship theories, implicit in the practice of infant observation, is the assumption that already in the early stages of the baby's development there is a relationship with the mother and with significant parts of her. Such a relationship correlates different experiences, possibly corresponding to different senses (Bion's 'consensuality'). The assumption that we are making is that one of the significant 'parts' to which the infant relates is the mother's mind.

This view, which is central to Bion's work, allows us to state our main point in concise terms: that wonder and delight at the discovery of the other's mind have an essential role in early development.

Our emotional experience when we discover another mind in adult life may be related to these early experiences. It is described by Keats in the sonnet 'On first looking into Chapman's Homer'. The poem, which he wrote after reading this beautiful translation ends with the lines:

Then felt I like some watcher of the skies
When a new planet swims into his ken;
Or like stout Cortez when with eagle eyes

He stared at the Pacific – and all his men
Look'd at each other with a wild surmise
Silent, upon a peak in Darien.

The way we are touched when we see babies exploring the world can also be understood as a reminiscence of our own infantile experiences. This process of discovery starts with the emotional link of knowing the other's mind. It is the basic relation which Bion called the K link (Bion 1962: 42–44). This chapter is particularly concerned with the prominent role of enquiry as a form of attention deployed both by mother and baby. We also noted that it can be constructively utilised by the infant to hold itself to things, and to good objects.

The columns of Bion's Grid correspond to categories used to describe the K link (Bion 1963: 17–20). Enquiry is one of the six categories he proposes. The mother's engaging of the baby's attention and the baby's lively response fall into another important Grid category, that of thought which effects development (Bion's column 6, action).

Yet another Grid category corresponds to the state of mind of the mother giving her attention to the baby in a receptive mood. She is receiving the baby's projections and is giving them a meaning. Bion called this the mother's reverie (Bion 1962: 34–36). For Vygotsky also, the mother uses the emotions she shares with the child to give meaning to the signs the child gives of his or her experience. The mother in turn would receive that meaning from her culture and from her own individual experience (Vygotsky 1960, 1984).

In the observations we discussed, the mothers' capacity for reverie was limited but the baby was the object of their constant concern. Together with love, this concern ensured that the baby was cared for. This in turn allowed the child to experience a modicum of thinking containment, even in the absence of reverie. The lack of reverie corresponds to the avoidance of emotional experience described by Bion as column 2 of the grid. (The remaining two Grid categories, those of notation and of definitory hypothesis, can also be recognised in the early relationship).

The K link is a link between two minds. This does not imply that the mother and her baby have a perfect or even a good understanding of each other. Misunderstandings frequently occur as, rather than reverie, the link is often that of attention given to the more sensuous manifestations of the other's mind. Also, avoidance of mental pain can result in a form of emotional blindness.

Emotional development depends on a capacity to tolerate both the mental pain of not reaching the other and the pain involved in linking to that other since the link might imply knowing the other's pain, anxiety or even hostility. Before anything else, however, such development relies on a determination to establish and sustain the relationship. In the first days of life, this determination may be in part innate. But it is also fostered by the other's attention.

The baby's interest in his mother seems to be the source of his interest in the world. As the poet Wordsworth was tracing his love of Nature to his first experiences he wrote:

> . . . blest the babe
> Nursed in his mother's arms, the babe who sleeps
> Upon his mother's breast, who, when his soul
> Claims manifest kindred with an earthly soul,
> Doth gather passion from his mother's eye.

We could add: blessed also the mother who gathers passion from her baby's eye.

What this chapter has attempted to show is that the passion one gathers from the other's eye is that of discovering the other's mind, with its rich promise of love and thought.

ACKNOWLEDGEMENTS

The first infant observation seminar of the Faculty of Psychology of the State University of Moscow developed from the efforts of Mrs Andrea Pound and Mrs Lynn Barnett to establish professional contacts between psychologists, psychotherapists and psychiatrists from Russia and Great Britain. With the help of Mrs Lynn Barnett and of Alex Dubinsky, Olga Bazhenova started this first seminar in October 1992. The interest and the contributions of the students were a constant inspiration. We were also helped by the comments and faithful support of Mrs Gianna Williams, Mrs Hélène Dubinsky, Mrs Margaret Goldwyn and Mrs Susan Keenes.

The British Council gave a travel grant to Olga Bazhenova to come to London to work on this chapter and attend the Tavistock Conference on Infant Observation, 1–4 September 1993.

REFERENCES

Bick, E. (1986) 'Further considerations of the function of the skin in early object relations – findings from infant observation integrated into child and adult analysis', *British Journal of Psychotherapy*, 2, 4: 292–299.

Bion, W. R. (1962) *Learning from Experience*, London: Heinemann.

Bion, W. R. (1963) *Elements of Psycho-Analysis*, London: Heinemann.

Bion, W. R. (1970) *Attention and Interpretation*, London: Heinemann.

Keats, J. (1944) 'On first looking into Chapman's Homer', in G. Bullett (ed.) *John Keats's Poems*, London: J.M. Dent and Sons.

Nikitina, G. M., Posikera, I. N. and Stroganova, T. A. (1987) 'Central organization of emotional reaction of infants' brains over the first year of life', in S. Trojan and A. Stastnj (eds) *Ontogenesis of the Brain, International Symposium*, 4: 223–227, Prague: University of Carolina Press.

Vygotsky, L. S. (1960) *Razvitie Visshikh Psykhicheskikh Funktsii* [The Development of Higher Mental Processes], Moscow: Izdatelsvo Academii Pedagogichesikh Nauk.

Vygotsky, L. S. (1984) 'Mladencheskii Vozrast' [The Age of Infancy], in D. B. Elkonin (ed.) *L.S. Vigotskii, Sobranie Sochinienii* [L. S. Vygotsky, Collected Works], 4: 269–317, Moscow: Pedagogika.

Wordsworth, W. (1985) 'The Two-part Prelude', in J. Wordsworth (ed.) *The Pedlar, Tintern Abbey and The Two-part Prelude*, Cambridge: Cambridge University Press.

Chapter 7

Thoughts on the containing process from the perspective of infant/mother relations

Pamela Berse Sorensen

In this chapter I am going to examine the component parts of the containing process. I hope that the reader has a basic familiarity with the work of Melanie Klein, Wilfred Bion and Donald Winnicott, since I am unable to elaborate my use of their work as a frame of reference within the limitations of this chapter. I use the phrase 'containing process' rather than the noun 'containment' in order to draw attention to its active rather than passive nature. In so doing, I wish to differentiate the concept of containment as I understand Bion (1962) to mean it, from the concept of the mirroring mother as used by Lacan (1977), Winnicott (1965) and Kohut (1977). I hope to explore, through vignettes from infant observation and child psychotherapy sessions, the complex, subtle and lively mental activity that contributes to, indeed constitutes, the work of a containing mind.

In using examples of ordinary mother/baby interaction parallel with material from psychotherapy sessions, I also wish to demonstrate that there are certain ways in which the work of the therapist serves to establish the possibility of a containing maternal mind which may be internalised by the patient and used as a vehicle for growth and development.

Let me be clear, I am not saying that the mother's work and the therapist's work are the same. There are many maternal tasks and functions which are obviously not therapeutic tasks or functions. Nor am I saying that containing is the *only* maternal function or the *only* therapeutic function. Clearly this is not the case. However, there is a state of mind or, more accurately, a way of thinking which is central to both; it is the elements of this way of thinking that I hope to identify and describe. These elements may come into play in any order or simultaneously.

OBSERVATION

The first such element and the basis for all the others is *observation itself.* This is fundamental to maternal mental work and the foundation of the containing process. Part of the enormous impact of having a baby is the sudden and overwhelming deluge of new and emotionally charged perceptions which impinge upon the mother. Where before a baby may have been large or small, pale or dark, cute or not, with the birth of her own baby suddenly every tiny detail of the baby's physical being becomes the focus of the mother's riveted attention. (I am speaking here in a normative sense. When Mother is uninterested or unobservant, we are worried, for we know that somehow keen observation is not only necessary for keeping the baby alive, but also the foundation of a loving relationship.)

The baby's tiny fingernails, a bit of crust on his scalp, or wax in his ear, a subtle change in his complexion or cry – these things become totally absorbing. This new wave of *passionate observation* may not be obvious to an outsider. Mother may be sitting still just 'being', in Winnicott's (1965) terms. But as we come closer, we see that she is scanning her baby's face and body in wonder, marvelling at how he is made. This is the beginning of her knowledge of him. And we may add, his experience of himself.

I am indebted to Dr Judith Sights for the following infant observation material. The observer met twice with Susan, a young mother in her twenties, before the birth of her second son. In these initial visits, Susan eagerly describes the active movement of the baby inside her and shows Judith ultrasound pictures and a video detailing the massive head, beating heart, liver, arms, legs, fist, penis and scrotum. The observer and Mother sit together on the couch looking at the pictures. Judith senses Mother's great longing to *know* the baby – the photographs are exciting, yet disappointing.

> The following week when Judith visits, the baby has been born. Mother ushers her into the bedroom where she lies down next to her sleeping newborn and pulls the blanket down away from his face. Mother is transfixed by the baby's face. She chats softly to the observer about baby Michael's startle response, his interest in light and dark shadows, his gentle hold on her finger, never taking her eyes from her sleeping baby's face. As he begins to stir, Mother says how funny baby noises are and gives examples of how he sounds in the early morning in the cradle, like a little animal. As his eyes flutter and open, mother begins talking softly and encouragingly to him. As soon as his eyes are open wider, she picks him up and deftly cradles him facing up for the observer to see. Noticing him grimace, Mother asks if he is hungry. She brushes his cheek with her finger in order to get him to turn to the right breast which, she confidently explains to Judith, is not his favourite. The observer says, 'The picture of him suckling at Susan's breast raised lots of powerful feelings in me: I'd always thought I didn't stare at nursing mothers out of respect for their modesty which may be partly true. But I also now realise it's because I cannot bear experiencing the beauty of the relationship in this most primary state. I want to be that baby, also to possess that baby, and finally to destroy that baby. I am

terrified by all of this, and it makes me want to look away. I got a quick glimpse of how I feel with patients at times when I am in tune with this part of them or we are in tune with each other: I get squirmy as if I can't stand this state of intimacy too much longer.'

What can we learn from this material about the containing process? Here I will use Bion's (1962) frame of reference of L, H and K links. First, I think we can see that Susan is operating under the influence not only of (L), that is, love for her baby, but also (K), derived from the first letter of the word knowledge, that is, the link between a subject which tries to know an object and an object which can be known. However, Bion assumes that the ultimate reality of the object is unknowable and therefore the Knowledge link necessarily carries with it some degree of frustration and pain. Where this emotional experience of frustration and pain can be tolerated, a modification occurs in which the imperfect knowledge acquired will be used to make further discoveries.

Where the experience of imperfect knowledge cannot be tolerated, the evasion of pain predominates and a −K or negative Knowledge link is generated in which meaning and emotion, discovery and development (of the mind) become impossible. Bion (1962) says that the negative Knowledge link substitutes morality for scientific thought. We could also add that −K substitutes clichés which masquerade as ideas. This may be a particular danger in our line of work.

From the beginning of her observations, the observer has impressed us with Mother's desire to learn everything she can about her baby. The technology of the sonogram leaves her thrilled and amazed but also disappointed, for it is the psychic reality of her baby she is after. Once he arrives, she becomes the scientist. She learns through all her senses the intricate details of his sucking, breathing, sleeping, visual preferences, responsiveness to sound and movement. She transforms these observations in the context of Love and Knowledge into the feeling which grows as time passes that she understands her baby much of the time.

Let us turn now to the observer's poignantly honest description of her own feelings as she witnesses the first feed. Envy has disturbed the Knowledge link in the observer. It is not tact which makes her turn away, but hate. She cannot continue her investigations because the force of beauty is too great and strains her generosity. It is better not to see, not to know. However, the observer is able to recover her capacity to bear this mental pain and in so doing a new and creative link is made between this pain of the present moment, envy at seeing the baby at the breast, and past difficulty in maintaining a Knowledge link with her patients. This is what Bion (1962) calls 'learning from experience'.

I would now like to turn to a consideration of our work as therapists and the role which observation plays in our ability to provide a containing experience for our patients. The containing mind is devoted to particulars. Read any account of a psychotherapeutic intervention which feels compelling in its truth and beauty and you will see that the same quality of rapt attention to detail prevails.

But why, one may ask, is this *dedication to dwelling in the particular* so important? Are we not wiser to let theory lead? After all, it represents the accumulated 'wisdom of the ages'. Is it not the theoretical and developmental models of the mind which ultimately offer the surest footing to both ourselves and our patients? An answer to this question is suggested by C. Fred Alford (1989: 153) in his book *Melanie Klein and Critical Social Theory*. In it he says that dwelling in the particular 'is about caring for the concrete suffering of real individuals. Individuals come before general ideas. It is for this reason that the details become so important.' In other words, dwelling in the particular represents the struggle to maintain a relationship to the object in the face of the pain of the unknown.

I would like to offer a description of a session with Bobby, a 15-year-old boy adopted at thirteen months and now living in a residential school for disturbed children. I am indebted to Dr Vanessa Camperlengo for this material.

> Bobby enters the room with a box. He is dressed, as always, in several layers of clothing with many pockets. He looks rumpled and baggy, his skinny arms and legs poking out of the clothes. Bobby sprawls in the chair and puts the box on the table. In it are many pieces of mechanical and electrical objects: springs, wires, batteries, screws and parts of a radio. None of these parts fit together. They are all in a jumble in the box. They are hard, metallic, small and sharp. Also in the box is a letter from his father. Bobby's nose is dirty. He doesn't use a tissue, though there is a box of them on the desk. He blows snotty, green bubbles from his nose and smears them on his sleeve. Taking a piece of fishing line from one of his pockets, he starts to floss his teeth. He flicks the gunk across the room. He takes a pair of scissors and starts to snip and then stab at the skin between his thumb and forefinger. He shaves the nail of his middle finger and picks at a hangnail. Bobby talks about the coming Thanksgiving holiday. He says he spoke to his mother on the phone. He hopes his parents will let him come home. Vanessa asks Bobby to put down the scissors. He begins to roll pieces of play-dough into balls and drops them on the floor. Then he cuts up tissue and lets it fall to floor. He picks up a battery, clenches it between his teeth and gives himself a shock by touching his tongue to the terminal.

At the end of this session, the therapist feels agitated and desperate. She is convinced that her therapy room is filthy with dirty scraps and asks me during supervision to help her clean it up. (The room in fact was not nearly as bad as she felt it to be.)

What Vanessa brought to bear in this session with Bobby was her willingness to notice every jagged, fragmented, painful manifestation of his experience of his world. She was able to allow the emotional quality of these manifestations to resonate within her and to sustain her Knowledge linking function sufficiently to bear active witness to each detail. This is the basic, fundamental, necessary beginning of the containing process.

Bobby nearly died of starvation as a baby. He was removed from his mentally retarded mother and then went to live with adoptive parents who withdrew from him when he proved to be unresponsive and unrewarding to look after. Bobby's psychic reality is filled with piercing, metallic fragmenting fear. Not only did he experience the unrelenting sharp torment of hunger, but even when this was relieved, he had little sense of being bound together through rapt attention to the particulars of his experience. He continues to feel in pieces.

However, he brings them in a *box*. And in this there is hope. For, I believe that the box represents not just the therapy as a place to put the pieces, but the hope that here his therapist will be of a mind to *notice exactly* what he has brought. And in so doing to gradually piece together an experience which has a meaning.

CLARIFICATION

The second component of the containing process is the work of clarification. By this I mean the effort to move, through some form of investigation, towards a more precise understanding of the nature of what has been observed. Mothers do this all the time. This is how Susan knew that baby Michael needed to start his feed on the right side rather than on the left, because she had noticed that he sucked more easily on the left and needed the incentive of hunger to get started on the right. Her clarification of his preferences allowed her to adapt her response to his inclination so that she could meet his nutritional needs and at the same time assuage his anxieties.

Such minute researches into everyday phenomena are so commonplace that we take them totally for granted. The 'environment mother' is indeed background. But the adaptations required to create this sense of background are the subtle, imaginative leaps of an actively inquiring mind.

For instance, one day at the dry cleaner's, I saw a mother working out how to soothe her crying toddler left alone in the car while she picked up her load of clean clothes. She couldn't take the toddler with her because she couldn't manage the clothes and baby. So she told the toddler that she could *see* her through the window the whole time and jockeyed herself into a position at the counter which enabled the baby to keep her eyes on her.

Perhaps on another day, this mother might just have been too tired or preoccupied with other things to have given much thought to the problem. 'Let the kid scream for two minutes, what the hell!' But in this particular interaction, this mother did feel able to investigate the baby's distress and was able to clarify for her that although she felt she was being abandoned when mother left the car she, in fact, was not, as could be demonstrated by seeing her and being seen by her.

The process of clarifying anxieties, sorting out one thing from another, differentiating, identifying, naming – these are mental activities which are part of the containing process. In Herbert Rosenfeld's 1952 paper, (in Spillius 1988: 37) 'Notes on the psychoanalysis of the superego conflict of an acute schizophrenic patient', his communications to the patient have the careful, one step at a time, simple quality of a mother patiently sorting out a terrible muddle.

> The patient sat silently on a chair, looking anxiously at the outside and inside of his hand. I asked, 'What are you afraid of?' He replied, 'I am afraid of everything.' I then said he was afraid of the world outside and inside, and of himself. He replied, 'Let's go back' which I took to mean that he wanted to understand the early infantile situation in the transference. He stretched out his hands towards me on the table and I pointed out that he was trying to direct his feelings towards me. He then touched the table tentatively, withdrew his hands and put them in his pockets, and leaned back in his chair. I said that he was afraid of his contact with me, who represented the external world, and that out of fear, he withdrew from the outer world. He listened carefully to what I said and again took his hands out of his pockets.

I hope that what is becoming clear is that when we talk of a containing object we are not talking about a passive receptacle for feeling, nor even simply a receptive space, but an active and responsive mind which is performing certain specific functions. Winnicott's (1965) evocation of the female element of 'being' as opposed to the male element of 'doing' in describing the prerequisites for successful containment is helpful in relieving us of certain misconceptions about therapeutic agency. But in emphasising the dichotomy between 'being' and 'doing' we may lose a sense of another mode which is neither the purely masculine element of doing nor the purely feminine element of being. This mode is active, but not in the sense of doing. It is active in the sense of focusing, discriminating and feeling. And ultimately *integrating* these functions in such a way that an experience, however fleeting, of containing and being contained is realised.

EMOTIONAL RESONANCE

I would now like to turn to the feeling part. Here I am talking about emotional resonance, an experience which is, perhaps, more chaotic, certainly less conscious than empathic perception. By emotional resonance I mean a deep and unconscious corresponding vibration within the internal object world – an experience of being open to the most primitive communication of the other. So much has been written about this in terms of the use of counter-transference as a therapeutic tool since Paula Heimann's 1950 paper on this subject. Our understanding of the mechanism of projective identification as a normal form of communication, which Bion first explored in his 1957 paper 'Attacks on linking' (first published 1959), has been elaborated and developed by many writers. Here I would like to offer two brief examples of what happens when the putative containing object is, for whatever reason, unable to allow a projection to resonate fully in the form of authentic counter-transference feeling.

The first is again, an example, from infant observation. I am grateful to Carolyn Johnson for this material.

> Baby Nathan (eleven weeks) is the second child and first son of a usually warm and affectionate South American mother. It is a rainy day. Mother is very tired and has a cold. She is uncharacteristically giggly and a little giddy on the day of this observation. Baby Nathan is lying on his back on a blanket on the floor. His movements are jerky and asymmetrical. Mother is sitting nearby eating some toast. When Nathan cries she picks him up and offers him the breast. He latches on, but after a few seconds he suddenly startles and throws his head back. Without hesitation, Mother stands up and gets a pacifier which the baby sucks on briefly and then rejects. Mother offers the other breast but Nathan cannot settle down. The observer feels tension between Mother and herself which she has never felt before. Mother, standing, bounces the baby vigorously up and down. His body seems stiff and his hands are in fists. His body relaxes a little, but he startles violently again then stiffens. Mother continues to bounce him and tells the observer that Nathan is fighting sleep and that she herself used to do this when she was a baby.

In this example, Mother is not able to allow the containing process to mobilise within her. She sees Nathan suddenly and violently pull back from the breast but she can neither investigate (try again, burp him, try the other side) nor allow his feeling of distress to distress her. She does two things. She plugs him up and passes on the distress to the observer.

The bouncing does not have the feeling of soothing, but rather the feeling of trying to *shake out* the bad experience. When Nathan startles and flings his head back again, mother substitutes an explanatory historical parallel for emotional resonance. At this moment, it seems, she cannot offer herself as an effective containing object.

This example is an ordinary bad moment in a bad day. Judging from previous observations, we have every reason to expect Mother to have a good night's sleep and recover her resources.

Less recoverable was my own capacity to bear the feeling of being with a borderline, adolescent girl whom I saw in a residential treatment setting once a week for nearly two years.

Jane, the only daughter and second child of a schizophrenic mother, had set fire to her family home when she was five. She had lived for several years with her very religious and puritanical grandparents who eventually could not tolerate her disruptive behaviour. She then was fostered by a well-meaning couple with a biological daughter Jane's age. The rivalry between the girls escalated to such a degree that Jane was removed from their home and placed in the special school where I saw her.

I dreaded Jane's sessions. I'd had experience with many severely deprived children in therapy over the years and was familiar with the sometimes long periods of hopelessness that must be endured during such treatments. But I had never felt so little capacity to sustain a sense of curiosity or a willingness to be used.

Jane flung herself into wild and extravagant demonstrations of her madness which left me unmoved. She would appear bedraggled and forlorn, then suddenly start snapping and eating her crayons – laughing and leering at me saying they were broken penises. She would begin describing an outing with the residential staff and the reporting would gather in momentum until it became a rapid barrage of senseless details about which I was both unable and unwilling to think. Pathetic one minute, vicious the next, her beautiful gray eyes would hang on mine and then suddenly she would be standing on the couch with her underpants down masturbating and cackling.

Jane would tolerate no remarks from me, but shouted me down, cruelly derisive of every attempt to talk to her about her experience.

Her treatment was a failure – a failure of basic containment. Jane smashed each tiny moment in which she might possibly have dwelled in my mind. I was not fast enough for her. An almost invisible beginning of a wish to communicate became a total and persecuting disaster when I could not understand her *instantly*. Then a calculated and cruel manipulation of her own madness would annihilate all hope of an effective containing mind by mocking integrity and sincerity itself. Everything became counterfeit. I felt that I was *playing* at being at therapist. I could observe. I could sometimes even puzzle over some things long enough to make some beginning clarifications, but the deeply integrating function of being open to projective identification lost the necessary vitality to sustain the treatment. I was relieved when it was over.

I was unable to contain for Jane what was most unbearable to her. I could not know it, resonate with it in my very being. Perhaps the reader may feel my disappointment and pain. This example may call to mind other failures of containment where that process which is so natural becomes remarkable by its absence or breakdown.

CONCLUSION

The containing process represents an active *integration* of observation, clarification and emotional resonance. No one function can alone provide the experience of containment. Observation alone may become the cold, clinical eye of a camera. Clarification alone may become arid formulation. Emotional resonance alone may become an idealised counter-transference which obfuscates the essential mystery and reality of the other.

Viewing the containment process as a struggle to integrate observation, clarification, and emotional resonance implies that we value the difficulty inherent in this task. This idea of *valuing difficulty* is a precious part of our psychoanalytic tradition and training culture.

In our work we are drawn close to the intimate struggles of patients and therapists, mothers and babies. At times we may become aware of great beauty in these struggles which comes, perhaps, from the creative effort involved in bringing together what we sense with what this may mean and what we feel about it.

REFERENCES

Alford, C. F. (1989) *Melanie Klein and Critical Social Theory*, New Haven, CT. and London: Yale University Press

Bion, W. R. (1959) 'Attacks on linking', *International Journal of Psycho-Analysis*, 40: 308–315.

Bion, W. R. (1962) *Learning from Experience*, London: Heinemann; reprinted in paperback, Maresfield Reprints, London: H. Karnac Books, 1984.

Heimann, P. (1950) 'On counter-transference', *International Journal of Psycho-Analysis*, 31: 81–84.

Klein, M. (1946) 'Notes on some schizoid mechanisms', reprinted in R. Money-Kyrle (ed.) *Melanie Klein: Envy and Gratitude and Other Works, 1946–1963*, Vol. 3, London: Hogarth, 1975.

Kohut, H. (1977) *The Restoration of the Self*, New York: International University Press.

Lacan, J. (1977) *Ecrits*, London: Tavistock.

Rosenfeld, H. (1952) 'Notes on the psychoanalysis of the superego conflict of an acute schizophrenic patient', *International Journal of Psycho-Analysis*, 33: 111–131; reprinted in E. Spillius (ed.) *Melanie Klein Today: Developments in Theory and Practice*, Vol. 1, London: Routledge, 1988.

Winnicott, D. W. (1965) *The Maturational Processes and the Facilitating Environ-ment*, London: Hogarth.
Winnicott, D. W. (1971) 'Creativity and its origins', in *Playing and Reality*, p. 80, London: Tavistock.

Chapter 8

Speculations on components in the infant's sense of agency

The sense of abundance and the capacity to think in parentheses

Anne Alvarez with Piera Furgiuele

INTRODUCTION

This chapter attempts to identify some components in what has been termed the infant's sense of agency. The normal infant is, in one way, helpless and dependent; but he is also competent, thoughtful, alert and, when conditions allow, full of passionate curiosity about his world. Developmental researchers have spent decades now in attempting to analyse the separate elements in the conditions essential for healthy cognitive/ emotional development. The sense of efficacy – or agency – is one such element identified by Broucek (1979). He has suggested that what he has called the 'sense of efficacy' – and the pleasure associated with it – are the foundations of self-feeling. In his book, (Broucek 1991) he cites Jonas, who thinks that the source of the concept of causality is in the experience of the body exerting itself in action (Jonas 1974). Broucek also describes Tompkins's observation that infants, soon after birth, 'replace reflex sucking with voluntary sucking and reflex visual tracking with voluntary visual tracking'. Tompkins apparently insists that from the first moments of life infants are engaged in making good scenes better by *doing it themselves* (Tompkins 1981). Broucek thinks this is one of the first manifestations of intent and of the will – a fascinating theory on the origins of basic self-feeling. Yet Broucek (1991) is clear that the infant is usually acting on some*one* and we might need to add, therefore, the equal importance of *object*-feeling – that is, feelings about the nature of the internalised human objects or representational figures which the baby sees himself acting upon. Clearly, causal experiences are not purely physical; they are also mental. The baby has plenty of experiences of his mind exerting itself in action and producing effects on another mind.

In the 1979 paper Broucek reviewed a number of research studies on 'contingency' (Broucek 1979). He described the baby's joyful delight in discovering that he himself can be a causal agent of events. The infant shows much pleasure – smiling, excitement and cooing – at the discovery that there is a contingent relationship between his own initially spontaneous behaviour and an event in the external world and 'the subsequent ability to produce *at will* the external event through repetition of the antecedent act. . . . The conclusion seems inescapable that the infant's pleasure in this situation is pleasure in being the cause.' He stressed the importance of the will – a relatively unexplored subject in psychology and in psychoanalysis and described what happens when babies are denied adequate opportunites for the experience of efficacy: if the baby is very young, the capacity for initiative may atrophy. Papousek and Papousek (1975), in a laboratory experiment, first gave babies the opportunity to cause an event to take place. The babies' pleasure was, apparently, insatiable. (The experiment showed that there was nothing special about the event itself that was rewarding – it was the ability to make it happen that mattered to the babies.) The experimenters then deprived the babies of this satisfaction, and found that the first reactions were intensified respiration, pulse rate and perspiration. However, an even more worrying situation arose: some of the babies began to 'play possum'; they lay motionless with non-converging, staring eyes and sleep-like respiration. Papousek and Papousek suggested that this passive state of a sort of 'total inner separation from the environment' was more likely to appear in babies under two months of age; infants older than three months placed in similarly frustrating situations seemed more able actively to avoid everything connected with the unsolvable problem. Active avoidance and passive unresponsiveness were thus seen as very different ways of reacting to a feeling of inefficacy; the result in both cases was a lowering of attention and orientation (Papousek and Papousek 1975). (There may be some interesting issues here for diagnostic and clinical consideration. Clinicians have considered it sometimes to be an achievement and a development when the withdrawal of an autistic child changes from being more automatic and helpless to being more actively intentional, when, for example, dull eyes are replaced by a deliberately averted gaze (Reid, personal communication; Alvarez 1992: 98)).

Psychoanalytic writers have discussed issues similar to, but slightly different from, the sense of agency or efficacy. Freud wrote of mastery (1920), Kohut (1985) of the need for self-objects. Melanie Klein made it clear that she distinguished between omnipotent defences and genuine potency in her *Narrative of a Child Analysis* (1961). Alvarez has stressed the danger for the therapist of confusing the child's triumph in his sense of omnipotence with his pleasure and shared pride in the sense of potency – and the importance of the latter in the recovery from certain types of severe depression in childhood (1992).

In his book which followed twelve years after the paper, Broucek (1991) makes it clear that the efficacy of the infant's efforts *vis-à-vis* the world depends on sensitive and 'good enough' maternal responsiveness. He had posited (1979): 'I cause and I intend, therefore I am', but he also points out that young babies are mostly interacting with human caregivers, not with the flashing lights of laboratory experiments. One might need, therefore, to expand his statement to read: 'I cause things to happen in her, therefore I begin to feel that I am, and I also begin to feel that she is.'

This chapter attempts to identify two possible components in this causal relationship. The first is the willingness of the caregiver to respond with thoughtful interest to the baby's initiatives and the baby's related sense of being a causal agent in evoking such responsiveness. This component concerns moments when the baby is in the foreground of the caregiver's interest, as implied in Broucek's argument. The first component (1) thus concerns a two-object relationship where the baby may feel a sense of agency toward one object. The second component, or rather, set of components (2) concerns a tripartite relationship, where the caregiver or baby is an agent in relation to two objects, and engages in something Jerome Bruner has called 'two-tracked thinking' (1968). Two slightly different behaviours of caregivers may help to facilitate the baby's development of this capacity.

The first (a) concerns the caregiver's capacity to keep the baby in the background of her mind at moments when some other object is in the foreground. It is possible that the baby's confidence in expecting this facilitates his consequent identification with an object capable of such two-tracked thinking.

The second behaviour (b) concerns the willingness of the caregiver to step aside *and wait* (interestedly) while the baby's attention is elsewhere. Thus, to repeat, in the first situation (as in Broucek's examples), the baby may experience agency in relation to one object; in 2a, he may experience himself as held in the back of someone's mind and so come to identify with that two-tracked capacity; in 2b, he may be able to experience agency in relation to two objects (one in the foreground, the other 'on hold' in the background).

In the three babies to be described below, both the first and second type of agency were seen to contain both emotional and cognitive features: first, the object acted upon was both responsive, reactive *and* interested mentally; second, emotional richness, a sense of abundance, in both the caregivers and the baby, was accompanied by an easy access to a wealth of ideas. A sense of the world's plenitude and replenishment seems to have connected with the feeling of being full of ideas – not ideas which crowd demandingly and confusedly for equal attention, but ideas which wait their turn in the queue but yet do not disappear. This may be related to what Bruner (1968) calls the capacity to 'think in parentheses', to manage two or more trains of thought at the same time. The three babies will serve to illustrate these phenomena. Alice, the first, and Angela, the third baby, were rich in both senses of agency; Paul, the second, was impoverished in both.

THE DEVELOPMENT OF TWO-TRACKED THINKING

Recently, Beverley Mack, an observer in a seminar at the Tavistock was impressed by an incident where Alice, a girl baby of one year and one week, had displayed a capacity for an interesting piece of two-tracked thinking. The observation took place on a day when the family's sitting room was full of people. Her very fond paternal grandparents were visiting, her father had returned from work, and her mother and 4-year-old brother Andrew were also present. At one point, in the middle of a peek-a-boo game, Alice fell over and hurt herself. Her mother comforted her, made her a drink and then carried her back into the sitting room:

> Mother sat next to Father and Alice sat enveloped by the contours of her mother's body, drinking her squash. She still had tears in her eyes and on her cheeks but was regaining her spirits. She sucked quietly at her drink and watched Andrew's activities. After a few minutes, Alice placed her cup on the ledge of Andrew's large toy car (almost the size of a large table), rested for a few minutes and – without looking – reached for the cup (accurately), grabbed it and began drinking again.

The observer was struck by Alice's capacity to remember, without looking, exactly where she had left the cup, while she seemed to be attending to something else. Another recent observation may serve to demonstrate the mindful attention both Father and Mother give to Alice. It also illustrates some interesting two-tracked thinking on the part of her mother, who showed a capacity to keep her in mind, just as Alice had kept the cup, while also attending to something else.

> Mother had placed a toy truck full of milk churns in front of Alice. The milk truck obscured my view but I think she removed a milk churn and put it in a little car. Father and Andrew then joined us. Mother noticed that Alice had a runny nose and wiped it. Alice moved her face sideways, as though trying to avoid being wiped. Mother then proudly said to Father that Alice can blow her nose and commented on how clever she is to be able to distinguish between her nose and mouth. Mother asked her to blow her nose, holding the tissue to her face. Alice smiled, obliged, and toddled off looking pleased with herself. Father said, 'She knows when she's being clever!' Alice continued to play, pushing her little car along the ground and following it, on her knees. She then removed another milk churn from the truck but dropped it, as Andrew caught her attention. Alice began to look around on the floor, seemingly in search of her milk churn. Mother, who had been in conversation with Father, suddenly said to Alice, 'Are you looking for your milk churn?' at which Alice got up and walked over to Mother.

Note how both Mother and Father underline Alice's new achievement;

Father then goes even further to show that he not only is interested in her clever new learning, he is interested in her state of mind *concerning* her cleverness. He knows she is being clever, but he also knows that she knows she is being clever (mental agency in the first sense). These are interested, responsive parents, but what particularly struck the observer as an additional element was Mother's capacity to know that Alice was looking for her milk churn, in spite of the fact that Mother's attention was on her husband at that point. She was able to keep her mind both on her husband and on her daughter. It did seem likely that Alice's impressive capacity to learn, and in particular, her capacity to manage two trains of thought at once, owed a lot both to her parents' capacity to lend her mindful attention when she was fully in the foreground of their minds, but also to their capacity, when other objects demanded their attention, to keep her in the 'back' of their minds (mental agency in the second sense).

Jerome Bruner (1968) has described a cognitive development which he has called the capacity to 'think in parentheses' or to hold something in reserve. It is fascinating to watch this capacity develop in previously mind-less psychotic and autistic children, and also in chronically depressed deprived children, as they begin to be able both to think and to believe in thinking. This achievement, however, is not purely cognitive and may bear some relation to the development in the infant of a phantasy or expectation of an available, enduring, even abundant world. That is, the infant's sense that I 'can do or have something', may be related to the sense that I 'am in the company of a do-able to or have-able object'; and even, perhaps, an object which will *wait* for me to have it fully or explore it fully and is, furthermore, content to wait – in brackets, as it were – while I interest myself in something else.

Bruner's strictly cognitive but fascinating study observed babies developing from a newborn state of one-tracked attention, where they can either only suck or only look, to a coordinated capacity for two-trackededness at four months, where they can do both more or less at once. (Early on, at the first stage, they shut their eyes while sucking; at the second stage, they begin to be able to alternate sucking with looking; at the third, they 'soft-pedal' the sucking, by engaging in non-nutritive sucking while they look at something. One imagines that this something is likely to be the mother's face!) Bruner (1968: 18–24, 52) calls this third stage 'place-holding', and describes an observation on the later move to threeness and to even greater conceptual multiplicity: the experimenter hands the infant one toy and then immediately hands him a second. *At about seven months*, the baby drops the first toy, picks up the second with the same hand, moves *it* to his mouth, and forgets the first. By about *twelve months*, the child is able to put the second toy in his free hand, but if he is offered a third, he drops one of the first two. He can manage two but not three. At about *a year and a half*, when offered the third, he no longer drops one, he puts one in the crook of his arm, so he has a free hand to take the third. He will then take more in the same manner. Bruner points out that the child has gone from a limit of one, defined by the mouth, to a limit of two, defined by the hands, to a limit of many, defined by a reserve.

Bruner does not discuss the conditions under which this sense of a reserve may be facilitated or hindered, but psychoanalysts have suggested that the move from two-person to three-person relationships may also play a part in the development of this type of deeper numeracy (Klein 1975; Britton 1989). Trevarthen's brilliant work (Trevarthen and Hubley 1978) on the developmental steps involved in the move from primary to secondary intersubjectivity – where the baby becomes able to take turns with his caregiver in playing with a toy – is relevant, too, although he, like Bruner, is less interested in the part the caregiver may play in facilitating these developments.

Clearly, as infant observation and infant research has shown, the relationship between the baby's mother and father, the degree of support for mother from grandparents, from internal figures, are all vital. An emotionally impoverished child, however, may be impoverished on the microcosmic as well as macrocosmic level, so we may also need to study very early and minute temporal patterns of interaction between mother and baby. How steady, for example, is the mother's gaze-holding while her young baby takes fleeting glances at her and away (Fogel 1977)? That is, how does the sense of a durable object get built up? How willing is the caregiver to follow the trajectory of the baby's gaze and to interest herself in his interests? For how many seconds can she sustain her interest in him *and* in his interests? Research has suggested conditions under which a baby's attention span to a single object may be prolonged (Stern 1977; Brazelton *et al.* 1974). One could speculate that the baby's paying attention to two objects at once (that is, to mother's background interest and the new object's foreground magnetism) may be facilitated by mother's ability to wait for the return of her baby's attention to her – that is, by her acceptance of his two-trackedness. He learns to accept her interest in other objects – father, siblings, household chores, the telephone – but she, too, learns to accept and respect his curiosity in things and people other than herself.

Bruner himself (1986), some years after this study, said that David Krech used to urge that people 'perfink' – perceive, feel and think at once. Urwin (1987) has criticised the cognitive researchers for seeing emotion as slowing down or speeding up cognition, whereas she, like the psychoanalyst Bion (1962), suggests that emotion enters into the structure of cognition itself. Can the sense of being able to hold something in reserve imply a mental phantasy of an object which will stay put, there in the crook of the arm of your mind, as it were? Will that toy or person or thought wait for you to get back to it? Or will it disappear? This capacity for holding firmly onto several strands of thoughts at one time must also depend to some extent on a prior phase – the one-tracked one, where each thought or experience is given time to be explored fully by both baby and caregiver. The will is, to a large extent, exercised on a willable – and perhaps willing – object. (It would be wrong, of course, to insist that the role of the actual caregiver is the only factor in this development. It is well established that some babies are born with a far greater capacity to shape their universe, and to hold their caregiver's attention, than others. However, it did seem that the two mothers of the two babies described below had very different notions of a reserve. Selection of material has meant some drastic over-simplification.)

Both babies, firstborns, were observed by female observers. They were observed for one hour a week at home with the major caregiver for a period of two years.

OBSERVATION OF PAUL

The parents of Paul were professional people in their middle thirties. Father and both sets of grandparents gave mother considerable support with the baby. During the first observation at home, Mrs J spoke at length to the observer about her anxiety and uncertainty about her capacity to be a good mother. She seemed sensitive and very concerned for her baby's well-being. At the week-two observation, she voiced a worry, common to many new mothers, as to whether she had enough milk. She added, without apparent awkwardness, that her sudden decision to supplement the breast feeds with bottles had probably been the result of her panic. This forgiving attitude to her own anxieties soon faded, unfortunately, and she began to be critical of everyone, including the baby, who dared to raise feelings of anxiety or failure in her. She could still be tender and affectionate when Paul's state of well-being gratified and reassured her, but at seventeen days, when the observer was certain that Paul was sucking contentedly at the breast, Mother said, uneasily, that he was 'only licking – only playing'. When she felt he was doing it again, she complained with some distaste of the hair in his ears. In later observations, she often warned him not to 'pull a face' when he was concentrating hard on sucking or defecating. When his lip drooped or his head lolled, she told him he was 'ugly'. We wondered who or what his perfectly ordinary and natural degree of infantile helplessness might have reminded her of. It was never clear.

Paul began to refuse to have the breast before the bottle and was weaned fully to the bottle at two and a half months. 'He turned his head away and there was nothing I could do about it', his mother told the observer disappointedly; then she added, 'It doesn't matter. It is even easier now. I am more free, because anyone can give the bottle to him.'

But there were signs that it did matter to this mother. It did affect her view of herself and make her even more critical. Paul, however, seemed determined to work hard to hold his mother's attention and to please her. He had a strong capacity to seek his mother's eyes, and to engage with her in a smiling way. She did at times respond to his loving communications deeply, but always fleetingly: she would suddenly cut off, look a bit lost, saying, 'What shall we do?' or 'What do you want?', as though the world which for a second had seemed full of possibility for both of them had suddenly emptied out. Her own belief in a object which could be of lasting interest seemed to be tragically impaired. In later months her sudden turning away became more active and decisive: she would simply go and make a phone call. She almost always held the baby facing away from her when she gave him his bottle, in spite of her own mother's pleas and protests about this.

When Paul was around three months, Mrs J seemed to harden up even more: she developed a sarcastic and at times cruel attitude to his by now slightly stronger vocal protests and greater bodily motility. The observer began to describe Paul as frequently being in a state of floppiness, with his eyes glazing over. He would begin to protest at being lain on his back in his pram for the umpteenth time, but he would quieten when he heard the icy threat in his mother's voice as she stared down at him and half held him down. What had started as a frightened inhibition on his part changed to a more listless apathy, as though he were giving up. In the seminar where the observations were discussed, we began to fear that Paul was in danger of a kind of psychic death.

By four months he had taken to biting his hands ferociously and trying to stuff toys all the way down his throat. An observation from four months and three weeks is fairly representative of much that followed in the months to come:

> When I arrive the atmosphere is tense; the mother says 'He is trouble-some because he has not slept this afternoon' (it is 18.15). Paul is pale, has rings around his eyes, a sad expression. He does not respond when I say hello. We go into the living room and his mother sits him on her knees, with his back to her, and at a distance from her. Paul tends to fall forward all floppy, saliva dribbles from his half-open mouth, his hands hang down. His look is a bit lost, eyes staring ahead. Every now and then he looks up to glance around and sometimes meets my eyes. He communicates deep depression. There is silence for a while. The mother is seated there and seems not to know what to do with the baby, with the time ahead of her, with me. Then a bit of conversation starts up. Mrs J indicates that she is dissatisfied with her husband who is not around enough, doesn't look after the plants on the balcony and doesn't share the housework with her. Paul gives out an 'iiih' of dis-

comfort. He moves a bit on his mother's knees, waving his little hands. His mother sits him down on the sofa beside her. 'He's not in a good mood because he has not slept much', she repeats. 'Then the afternoon becomes long, and he gets bored. . . . It's not time for your feed until a quarter to eight', she says, turning to the baby who has uttered another 'iiih'. She continues to talk to me; I listen with attention, keeping an eye on the baby. She says that yesterday they visited a friend who had just had twin girls. She is disappointed that Paul spent the whole time with some red cloth pot-holders instead of getting interested in the babies; she wanted him to get to know them, as they would be going to nursery school together. Paul starts uttering his 'iiih' again. He moves a little on the sofa. 'I wonder what he wants to say to us', I say. 'Nothing', replies his mother, 'He is just troublesome because he hasn't slept.' The baby gives out a louder 'iiih'. 'Here it is, this is the new thing he learnt two days ago, he has learnt to squeak!' comments his mother sniggering. Paul, who has been turning his head every now and then to look at me, now stares at me for a long time. I smile at him and say, 'Hello Paul.' He continues to look at me. I have the clear sensation that he is waiting for me to speak to him again. I feel in a difficult position. I smile again. I say a few words to him. Paul looks at me again for a moment, then he turns towards his mother and says 'Eh! eh!', waving his little hands. 'Yes, eh?', echoes his mother, 'What do you want to say? Eh? Aren't you comfortable? Shall we change position?' She sits him down in the corner of the sofa and looks at him in silence for a while. Paul has slipped down into a hunched position. His mother laughs and pulls him up. 'Do you know that he has nightmares now?' she adds, in a rather worldly tone. 'Last night he woke up twice. . . . The best thing is to leave him there with his dummy. . . . Perhaps he ate too much and didn't digest it properly.'

It was very painful for the observer and the seminar group to witness this mother's depression, cynicism, and her difficulties in seeing Paul's needs. Paul needed desperately to be entertained. He wanted attention, some conversation, some play. But Mrs J felt empty and at a loss. She seemed not to be able to believe that she herself could be the main object of interest – and one of lasting interest – for the baby. She ended up actively preventing Paul from remaining in contact with her. She held him with his back to her and seemed unaware of his struggle to regain her face, her eyes, her attention. The observer's comment, aimed at helping to re-establish communication, went unheeded. The mother felt disappointed and irritated, became sarcastic and minimised and mocked the baby's achievement (his 'squeak'). After a moment, perhaps helped by the fact that the baby's call had a different quality, and conveyed more life and interest to her, and perhaps because she has been able to identify a little with the observer's 'conversation' with the baby, the mother was able to be kinder to Paul: she wanted to seat him more comfortably. She looked after him for a while, mentioned his nightmares.

However, later in the same observation, Mother was speaking to the observer about the fact that chatting with Paul was amusing, he seemed to reply nowadays, there were real dialogues:

> She is interrupted by shrill 'iii' from Paul, who has become hunched in the corner of the sofa and is slipping down. Mother makes an impatient gesture. 'What do you want, eh? what do you want?' she asks in a harsh tone, 'Let's have a bath, shall we? eh? Is that what you want? Shall I give you a lovely bath?' The tone is falsely kind and jokey; it contains a hard note of threat. The baby falls silent. His mother says to me, laughing, 'The bath terrorises him. He is scared stiff', and something else that I miss because I am too preoccupied with my feelings. Paul utters a feeble lament. His mother says, 'Do you want to look at your hands? Come on, look at your hands a while.' She explains to me that he has learned to put his thumb in his mouth, sometimes both of them together. The baby in fact is doing this. His mother comments, 'Oh what a comfort! What a comfort your thumb is! You have two, you can suck one and then the other!' Paul, with his thumb in his mouth, tries to turn round towards his mother. He doesn't succeed, makes a sound of protest and waves his arms and legs in an attempt to move himself as he wants; he whines, rubs his eyes and bursts out crying. 'What do you want?' says his mother, 'Are you inconsolable? Come on, let's sit like this.' She sits him down again properly on her knee, with his back to her, she puts his hands on his legs where he can see them and crosses her hands over Paul's tummy so as to keep him still. When Paul tries to move she applies pressure to his tummy with her hands. The baby stops trying almost immediately, is silent, stares ahead. His look becomes dull and blank. 'Is it better like this? You always calm down when I put you like this, don't you?' his mother says to him.

This material is almost unbearable to read. Paul's mother wants a lively intelligent baby, but cannot resist discouraging his initiatives. She rejects his interest in her, and almost forces him into physical immobility and mental emptiness. The result seems to be a terrible loss of initiative and efficacy, a kind of sapping of his will. During the whole observation a depressed and persecutory atmosphere hung in the air, making it very difficult for the mother to do the right things and for the observer to be of help. The observer felt that anything – silence, words, doing, not-doing – could be felt as persecuting and thus rejected or devalued. It was very painful for the observer to see Paul's dazed expression, and this mother make efforts to find a way into her baby, fail, and then seem to harden herself. This led to even more disdainful and even cruel behaviours with the baby, in which she often sought the observer's collusion. The observer sometimes felt a mute request in the sad expression of the baby to which, in her role as observer, and in the light of mother's competitiveness and touchiness, she could respond in only minimal ways. She tried, in a variety of tactful ways, to help this depressed but also narcissistic and controlling mother to get together with her baby, including, when even Mother eventually acknowledged concern about Paul's mental development, suggestions about where she could get information and help. But these were rejected. We were aware that Paul was losing his will to make an impact on his world, but we began to fear that he would lose his mind, too.

Yet all was not lost. Mrs J sometimes seemed able to get relief from the fact that someone else, in her presence, was looking after the baby and the relationship with Paul was therefore mediated at some distance. The baby seemed a little happier, too. In the same observation, for example, we see things going better with the arrival of the father.

> At first the father speaks with the mother, and the baby, left to himself, leans forward with a sad dazed look and with saliva dripping down. Then the father picks him up, walks with him and talks to him. He sings him nursery rhymes which he usually makes up specially for him. Paul seems to start to feel that he exists again; he comes back to life, says 'ghee'. Little by little, he begins to explore his surroundings with his eyes again. The mother is now more relaxed. She smiles at him from the sofa and says 'Hello' in a loving tone. After an initial moment, when he refuses to look at her, encouraged by his father, Paul turns and smiles back. The mother is content and greets him again. The father is relieved and exclaims 'Oh, there, a smile at last!'

Similar recoveries were observed when the grandmother was present. Unfortunately, although there were two parents present for Paul at this moment, there was rarely little sense that both were fully present for him. At least during such episodes with his father or a grandparent, he had, finally, the care of one, with his mother as a not unfriendly witness. Such threeness as existed was a pale shadow of what we shall see in the next observation. Mother's personality difficulties seemed to have been profound and the help of relatives did little to reduce her cynicism and boredom. She soon began to look back with regret on her former life. She complained that 'It is no fun' being a mother and that she could do it only 'in small doses'. Mothering was devalued and Paul often referred to as a little animal (frog, tortoise) as though he were without needs or feelings and therefore capable of being left to his own devices for long periods. Not long after the reported observation he began to resort to repetitive bouncing up and down in a sort of muscular self-containment and his biting of his hands worsened. He began beating himself. He was often placed on the floor to play alone, and here he engaged in activites of an ominously repetitive quality; he would sit and simply shake a toy monotonously. He also had many moments of immobility and passivity.

At seven months, Mother's anxious but bullying need to control and limit Paul's inititatives extended to his attempts to handle his feeding cup, and also to his tentative attempts at physical adventure and exploration. She complained that he was at the bottom of the class developmentally and tried to 'teach' him to roll over. (Most babies teach themselves to roll over because the world beckons from the other side. Paul had relatively little to strive for and, anyway, little belief in his own capacity to get it.) His mother interpreted his reaching for a bright red cube in a tower she set up for him only as a wish to knock it over. She was often frustrated by his apathy, but could not help engendering it. Any sense of himself as an active agent in his world seemed terribly impaired. In many ways, he seemed to have given up on such ideas. He was becoming a little Oblomov.

Yet at around nine months, after a family holiday and some improve- ment in Paul's motor skills and in his ability to understand (or rather in his mother's belief that he understood), Mrs J did seem somewhat more interested in him – as a sort of little pupil. Her husband was helpful and easier with Paul than was she, but he was very busy himself, and they tended to take turns in his care, rather than being together with him. Also, Father, like the grandparents, treated his fragile but demanding wife with great caution and never crossed her. In fact, they all seemed afraid of her. On one occasion when Paul was sixteen months, he indicated that he wished to get close to some flowers in the sitting room. Mother took him to them in her arms, insisting, 'Don't touch, just look!' and then immedi- ately tried to get him to name the colour of the bright yellow mimosa flower. As usual, she was bent on pulling from him the response she wanted, rather than respecting his spontaneous, but as usual, only very gently demanding, request. When he did manage, at the next vase, to reach out and touch a peach blossom and inadvertently to knock one off, she said, 'Don't knock all the flowers off – the bare twigs will be so ugly!' There is, possibly, a glimpse here of what may have lain behind her cruelty and hard impatience. The world was unreplenishable. There was no reserve: it really seemed as though she felt there could never be more peach blossoms ever again in the universe. At this stage, she could not let herself be a patient witness to Paul's explorations: she either interfered impatiently, or abandoned him to it to get on with it himself.

Soon after her return to work, however, she became somewhat more animated and able to enjoy some of Paul's independent explorations around the house. For example, she did permit him to take books off the shelf and look at them. She liked 'teaching' him and he mostly did learn to name things, always looking up immediately to her for praise. She worked hard to make him numerate. There may be a painful lesson here in the difference between numeracy and the sense of a deeper multiplicity and of a something available in reserve, of a replenishable abundant universe. (When the observer had given Paul a toy elephant as a gift for his first birthday, Mother had said dismissively 'He's already got two.') Abundance from others, like the support of her parents and of her husband which she could never acknowledge except with contempt, seemed not to enrich her; it threatened her autonomy or else was beneath her notice.

Yet it was clear that Paul had managed to emerge from his previous listlessness and had not become severely withdrawn. He had found a way through to his mother and she to him, up to a point. It was hard to find evidence that he ever learned much for its own sake or for his own. By now, he was almost always on the move, and his anxieties at times were overwhelming. He was regularly distraught when his mother would sneak out to work. He would grab desperately for his cup at mealtimes, as though he could not believe it was really coming toward him and would be his for a while. We never heard of the kind of exploratory play that we shall hear of in the next baby. And there was certainly little time for reflection.

When sent to a day nursery, at ten and half months, he was so anguished and so often physically ill that the nursery staff felt he could not stand it and begged his mother to keep him at home. She refused. But, as indicated, Paul did find a way through, however narrow and single-tracked its quality: he did learn to name objects and to count, and he did work hard to please. Although he clearly benefited considerably from the care of his loving grandparents, he did not seem to feel rich and blessed in the sense of feeling he had, as did the next baby, many loving caretakers. Rather, like the rest of his family, all of whom seemed both to idealise and fear (and possibly fear for) his mother, Paul behaved much of the time as though there was really *only one* very powerful object in his inner world, and that it was indeed a precariously available and quite dangerous one. Safety, when it arrived, was also precarious and short-lived, and never durable enough to see him through separations, or even through a period of exploratory play. There was no sign of the relaxed, playful reflectiveness we shall see in the next baby.

It is also true that on the more microcosmic level of brief second-by-second encounters, his mother did not wait for Paul to complete an engagement with her or with a toy; nor, however, did she wait and watch with interest when his interest shifted to something or someone else. She took it as an opportunity to escape. Paul seemed to be developing with an impaired belief in the durability of his object's existence and in his own ability to prolong its stay or to bring it back when it was absent. There were many signs, in the limited and careful quality of his play, that, in addition to the obvious effect on his confidence and his emotional life, there was also impairment in his cognitive capacities. His anxieties seemed to make all activities, except the most cautious of ones, short-lived and lacking in potential for development (see Murray 1991, on the effect of maternal post-natal depression on infant and child cognition).

We shall give a much briefer report of the third baby, and are grateful to Dr Pia Massaglia for permission to use this material.

OBSERVATION OF ANGELA

Angela was born to parents who told the observer that they worked in a factory. Much later, she learned that they were engineers. In the hospital, when Angela was three days old, Mother told the observer that she had noticed that Angela alternated smiles with frowns: 'She goes from beautiful thoughts to horrible ones in the space of a second.' At home, Father commented on the baby being nervous, and mused about the idea that their house must be very different from the hospital for her. He 'hoped she would get the hang of it!' Note that the baby already is seen as having thoughts, feelings, and acute sensitivities – the very sensitivities and lability to which a very new baby is indeed prone. And the parents seem to have the sense already that *things take time*. This mother, like Paul's, also had anxieties about whether she had sufficient milk, and was for a time quite obsessional about cleanliness and feed times; but in the second week said that she had learned that the baby's noises and stretches at night did not indicate dissatisfaction, so she had been able to stop checking on her all the time. Also, she said that she thought the baby followed her more with her eyes now. We can note this mother's capacity to be reassured, and the pride in learning something about her baby, and also the sense of respect for the baby's agency and competence, and for her own. Already there are at least two figures in the picture, each with some recognisable space and competence of her own.

At thirty-five days Mother described how Angela did not seem able to grasp the rattle on her own but could hold it if mother helped by putting it into her hand. At one point she said to Angela, 'You like your friend the pendulum clock, don't you!' and then turned Angela so that she could see it better. At a feed in a later observation, Mother showed some irritation and jealousy of the baby's interest in, and seeming preference for her pendulum 'friend' over finishing the first course of her meal, but accepted defeat, did not insist the baby finish, and offered some different, possibly more enticing food, instead. A compromise offers a third option to two warring factions. A mother who waits while you express an interest in something else is remaining in reserve in a very significant way, and this is an emotional, but perhaps a cognitive experience too. We learned that Mother could also accept Angela's more active protests. At four and a half months Mother remarked to the observer that Angela had begun to notice that she could pass something from one hand to the other! In fact, Angela became a very advanced baby.

It needs to be added that the sense of resources in reserve was very much present in both sets of Angela's grandparents and in her father, all of whom were patient but not indulgent with the child. At six months, when Mother was soon to start working again, and Maternal Grandmother would become the regular childminder, she offered Maternal Grandmother the opportunity to feed fruit to the baby. The grandmother replied, 'You give it to her, I'll have lots of time.' At eight months, Mother tried to show Angela that her new toy train moved. Then she commented, 'You're not interested in its movement, you've found out it makes a noise. It's your toy, use it how you want.' The observer noted that Angela, who was a thriving and lively baby – little has been said about her personality, in order to concentrate on the the cognitive/emotional elements – had what psychologists call the 'extension concept' and was able to pull a sheet to get a remote toy which was lying on the sheet. Angela's parents were often together with her, and both of them were tremendously interested in her. For them it seemed that the world was interesting and *her* world was interesting. At just under ten months, Father told the observer that: 'When Angela holds the plastic keys in one hand, she immediately puts them in the other hand, then she shows the empty hand, and keeps the keys!' (He smiled at the last phrase.)

SUMMARY

These three observations have been used to illustrate two possible elements in the sense of agency: the sense of mental agency in relation to one object; and the sense of mental agency in relation to two objects. The latter has been linked with Bruner's concept of the sense of a reserve (1968). The material from the first baby, Alice, illustrates the capacity of the parents to provide opportunities for both foreground mindfulness (1) and background mindfulness (2a); it also illustrates the existence of related developments in the capacity for two-tracked thinking in Alice herself. Paul's experience and development seems to have been impaired in both respects. The material of Angela, the third baby, was rich in 1 (mindfulness in her objects and in herself) and in 2b (the sense of an object which can wait for your return). The sense of a reserve has been linked with the sense of agency, and the chapter has suggested some emotional elements which may be significant for this apparently cognitive development. Emotional and cognitive impoverishment in one baby has been contrasted with a sense of multiplicity, plenitude and the apparent development of complex 'thinking in parentheses' in two others. Perhaps agency and intelligence are linked, and perhaps both are linked with an intelligible caregiver who feels that both the infant and his interests are intelligible and worth waiting for.

ACKNOWLEDGEMENTS

We are grateful to Dr Pia Massaglia of the Department of Child Neuropsychiatry, University of Turin, and Beverley Mack of the Tavistock Observation Course for their assistance.

REFERENCES

Alvarez, A. (1992) *Live Company: Psychoanalytic Psychotherapy with Autistic, Borderline, Deprived and Abused Children*, London: Routledge.

Bion, W. R. (1962) *Learning from Experience*, London: Heinemann.

Brazelton, T. B., Koslowski B. and Main, M. (1974) 'The origins of reciprocity: the early mother–infant interaction', in M. Lewis and L. A. Rosenblum (eds) *The Effect of the Infant on its Caregivers*, London: Wiley Interscience.

Britton, R. (1989) 'The missing link: parental sexuality in the Oedipus complex', in *The Oedipus Complex Today: Clinical Implications*, London: Karnac.

Broucek, F. J. (1979) 'Efficacy in infancy: a review of some experimental studies and their possible implications for clinical theory', *International Journal of Psychoanalysis*, 60: 311–316.

Broucek, F. J. (1991) *Shame and the Self*, London: Guilford.

Bruner, J. S. (1968) *Processes of Cognitive Growth: Infancy*, Worcester, MA.: Clark University Press

Bruner, J. S. (1986) *Actual Minds, Possible Worlds*, Cambridge, MA.: Harvard University Press.

Fogel, A. (1977) 'Temporal organization in mother–infant face-to-face interaction', in H. R. Schaffer (ed.) *Studies in Mother–Infant Interaction*, London: Academic Press.

Freud, S. (1920) 'Beyond the pleasure principle', *Standard Edition 18*, London: Hogarth.

Jonas, H. (1974) *Philosophical Essays* New York: Prentice Hall.

Klein, M. (1961) *Narrative of a Child Analysis*, London: Hogarth.

Klein, M. (1975) 'The role of the school in the libidinal development of the child', in *Love, Guilt and Reparation and other Works*, London: Hogarth (first published 1923).

Kohut, H. (1985) *The Analysis of the Self*, New York: International University Press.

Murray, L. (1991) 'The impact of post-natal depression on infant development', *Journal of Child Psychology and Psychiatry*, 33: 543–561.

Papousek, H. and Papousek, M. (1975) 'Cognitive aspects of preverbal social interaction between human infants and adults', in *CIBA Foundation Symposium*, New York: Association of Scientific Publishers.

Reid, Susan (personal communication)

Stern, D. (1977) 'Missteps in the dance', in *The First Relationship: Infant and Mother*, Cambridge, MA.: Harvard University Press.

Tompkins, S. (1981) 'The quest for primary motives: biography and autobiography of an idea,' *Journal of Personality and Social Psychology*, 41: 306–329.

Trevarthen, C. and Hubley, P. (1978) 'Secondary intersubjectivity: confidence, confiding and acts of meaning in the first year', in A. Lock (ed.) *Action, Gesture and Symbol: The Emergence of Language*, London: Academic Press.

Urwin, C. (1987) 'Developmental psychology and psychoanalysis: splitting the difference', in M. Richards and P. Light (eds) *Children in Social Worlds*, Cambridge: Polity.

Chapter 9

Psychosomatic integrations
Eye and mouth in infant observation

Maria Rhode

INTRODUCTION

The shorthand term, 'breast', has long been used in psychoanalytic writing to denote the totality of what the mother provides for her baby: love, warmth, understanding, interest and stimulation as well as food (Klein 1952). Therapy with autistic children has demonstrated the crucial import-ance for ongoing development of a proper use and integration of the various senses (Meltzer *et al.*, 1975; Tustin 1981); while work by develop-mental psychologists (Stern 1985) shows that the normal young baby is capable of the cross-modal transfer of patterned information and of evolving internal representations of a higher level of abstraction that are not tied to a given sensory mode.

Among psychoanalytic authors, Spitz (1955) and Winnicott (1967) first pointed to the importance of eye contact between mother and baby. Interest is now focusing on tracing in detail how the senses interact and what can interfere with this. Haag (1991), Reid (1990), Wright (1991), Pines (1993) and, in this volume, Maiello, have all made recent contributions in this area.

This chapter explores the integration between mind and body in the mother–baby relationship: a rough equivalence is proposed between mind and eye contact on the one hand, and body and mouth contact on the other.

A post-autistic 5-year-old patient of mine brought along to a session a miniature cheese with a red wax coating, which he proceeded to peel off. After eating the cheese, he held the torn coating up to his eyes, then exchanged it for the translucent red plastic envelope for his scissors. Pre-viously he had cut bits out of this envelope; now he used it as 'blood-coloured' glasses through which he looked at the world. This child could not assume a sense of agency: owning a sense of himself would have meant attributing to his own oral sadism the bleeding internal objects he apprehended in his mother's face. She had in fact been deeply depressed when he was born.

When he came to treatment, this boy showed the gaze avoidance typical of the autistic and post-autistic child. Material like that of the blood-coloured glasses made it more than understandable to me that he should use autistic devices to blot out the meaning he might otherwise fear to see in my eyes. Much later in his treatment, incidentally, when eye contact had become possible, he sang over and over again the words of a pop song, 'Look into my eyes'.

Experiences such as this have made me wonder how often the pathological over-emphasis on sensation at the expense of meaning, that we come across in autistic children as well as in psychosomatic symptoms, in fact may follow from an apprehension that the meaning would be intolerable. This would link with work on psychosomatic reactions by Joyce McDougall (1989) as well as by Kleinian authors (for example, S. Klein 1965, 1980). It would go against the view that in the beginning is bodily sensation and that mind gradually evolves out of this – a view widely held since Freud's famous statement in *The Ego and the Id* (1923) that 'the ego is first and foremost a body ego'.

Until the recent flowering of research on the capacities of very young infants, it could be tempting to think of bodily experience 'developing' into mental, particularly when the theory of alpha function (Bion 1962) might be interpreted as providing a model for such a process. However, besides tracing the evolution of infants' capacities, researchers have now documented the very considerable competence present in the newborn, which can involve the interplay of different sensory modes (see, for instance, Stern 1985) and the unlearned capacity for cross-modal transfer (Meltzoff and Barton 1979). Negri (1994) has reported that sensory stimulation in a ten-day-old baby triggers a visual search for the source of the stimulus. Clearly it is necessary to follow through on the theoretical implications, and to refine formulations concerning the growth of mind out of bodily experience or the development of sensation into emotion (see Tustin 1994).

If one turns to infant observation for answers to the question of how psyche and soma interrelate in the course of so-called normal development, one is struck by two very commonplace facts. The first is that, when things are going well, mothers talk about their babies as though they were human beings, not members of a different race called 'babies'. Mothers may sometimes be apologetic about this, as though they expected the observer to criticise them; but by and large, if mothers talk about their babies as though they belonged to a different species, we take this as a sign of a hitch in communication. (Probably even the most ardent follower of William James or proponent of the importance of nerve tract myelination would in practice have reacted much as we do: he would have expected mothers to attribute personalities to their tiny babies even if he had thought them misguided.) A parallel process, incidentally, tends to go on in the seminar. Once the observers begin to take for granted that the baby is expressing human feelings, though in an unfamiliar way, the strangeness of detailed observations ceases to be a problem.

The second, and related, fact is that a mother will interact with her baby *as a person* at the same time as she cares for his body. For example, imagine a young baby on his mother's lap, in a relatively unintegrated state, perhaps not focusing on anything in particular, moving his arms and legs in an uncoordinated way. A mother's ordinary response will probably involve at least three components: she may look at the baby, take his hand in hers or bring her hand up to meet his foot, and perhaps say something like, 'What are you looking for?' or 'Here I am' or 'What's the matter?' My point is that a commonplace hypothetical event like this one illustrates the way in which the attribution of meaning is brought together with the definition of the baby's body as well as with a visual encounter. In other words, mental and physical experience come together: *and in the first instance, this must happen in the mother's mind.* (I hope to show later that the baby has a preconception of an object that is both integrated and integrating, not just with regard to 'common sense', but with regard to sensory and emotional experience.) If mental and physical experience come together consistently enough, we could expect our hypothetical baby to grow up possessing what an obsessional patient in a recent paper by Ryz (1993) felt that he lacked: 'A bridge between the feelings in my stomach and the thoughts in my head.' For this to be so, the mother will need the capacity to see her baby as a separate person; the baby will need to be able to accept what the mother offers.

We are dealing here with that function of the environment (for babies, of the mother), that group analysts, in particular, have called 'mirroring'. This is the function by which someone outside us responds to our being and 'reflects' it back to us in such a way as to make us aware of ourselves in terms of the effect we have produced (Pines 1987). Winnicott described the visual component of this process in 'The mirror-role of mother and family in child development', within the framework of his theories of early omnipotence and environmental failure (Winnicott 1971). My aim here is to emphasise the simultaneous interplay of the different modes of experience in the example of a hypothetical baby.

On a bodily level, the baby's hand or foot is coming up against his mother's hand, the presence of which is delineating his boundaries. On a mental and emotional level, by means of her interest and attention, she is offering herself as someone who attributes meaning and intentionality to his behaviour. At a deeper level, this will be linked with alpha-function. An essential aspect of the mother's contribution is that it is transformatory rather than mechanically reflective. Alvarez (1992) has emphasised this point in considering the importance of the mother's liveliness.

I wish to suggest that when the balance of these interacting modes is disturbed, so that the harmonious interplay between them is blocked, we can observe the integration of sensation and meaning being interfered with. I propose that this integration of sensation and meaning is illustrated by the interplay of eye contact and mouth contact between mother and baby. As far as I am aware, it is only relatively recently that analytic writers have taken a systematic interest in the implications of eye contact for infant development, and particularly in its interaction with other modes. (I am thinking of such authors as Haag 1984, 1991, 1992; Reid 1990; Wright 1991; Pines 1993). Spitz is an important exception: he emphasised forty years ago that a feeding baby looks into his mother's face rather than at the breast (Spitz 1955). Tustin (1981) has written about vision as the sense that acknowledges spatial separateness, while Bion (1950) has linked binocular coordination to the integration of the primal couple. Meltzer (1986) has discussed the 'eye as nipple', that is, as an object of Oedipal jealousy, and also the eye as representing the earliest superego. With his colleagues (Meltzer *et al.* 1975), he has pointed to the dismantling that 'common sense', which of course includes vision, undergoes in autism.

Geneviève Haag reviews the tradition within French psychoanalysis of emphasising the interplay between touch and vision (Haag 1992). She sees the 'jump into the mother's eyes' ('*le saut dans les yeux*'), associated with benign projective identification, as the necessary condition for overcoming the infant's terror of falling through space and the constant reliance on sticking to the surface of people or things (adhesive identification, Bick 1968). The balanced interplay between the interpenetration of nipple and mouth on the one hand and the eyes on the other is seen as underlying bodily integration, particularly the proper experience of the joints (Haag 1991).

What I wish to propose, then, is a very rough correspondence between eye contact and meaning on the one hand, and mouth contact and sensation on the other. When Bion says, 'milk, we may assume . . . is received and dealt with by the alimentary canal; what receives and deals with the love?' (Bion, 1962: 33) he is referring to the whole of the infant's developing psyche-soma. I am suggesting here only that the love – or absence of it – is received by the eye, whatever those structures may be that allow the love to be recognised as a realisation of the infant's preconceptions. As W.B. Yeats put it, 'Wine comes in at the mouth/And love comes in at the eye' (1910).[1]

I will now pass to material from infant observations. The first observation provides evidence for the baby's preconception of what I shall call an integrated object, that is, one in relation to which emotional and bodily experience, eye and mouth, can come together. The second observation illustrates the disjunction between eye and mouth, accompanied by soma-tisation, occurring after a separation the meaning of which mother was not able to acknowledge. In the third, we see how a similar disjunction, with compensatory emphasis on the physical provision of food, could be healed thanks to the presence of an observer who was receptive to emotional communication.

BABY ARTHUR: THE PRECONCEPTION OF AN INTEGRATED OBJECT

Arthur was his parents' first child, and was five weeks old at the time the visits began. The observer noted that Arthur's mother was concerned not to pick him up too soon 'in case he got used to it', and that she seemed to be doing things by the clock:

> The baby seemed frightened most of the time, grimacing and clenching his fists apart from when he was breast-feeding, when he would appear to be in a different world, silent, eyes closed and peaceful.

The breast is a refuge from frightening emotions, experienced in sensual terms, without eye contact. There is an impulse towards differentiation however:

> I noticed in the first two observations that Arthur's ability to focus with his eyes had improved and that on the second visit he looked straight at me for some time.

> At seven and a half weeks, Arthur was smiling and relaxed. He had a quick and peaceful feed during which his eyes were shut and he retained the nipple in his mouth even after he had stopped sucking. His mother said that this was usual. When she changed his nappy, Mother spent a good ten minutes cooing at him. He seemed to love it and responded by gurgling and smiling and lifting and dropping his arms and legs. There was a strong communication going on and this was the first time that I had seen it. It was wonderful to observe. I also thought that her attitude towards Arthur was very different here. She was totally with him.

The observer speculated that Mother had been encouraged by comparing Arthur favourably with another baby. This contrast between the emotional contact during feeding and changing persisted as a feature of the observations.

> Between this visit and one at twelve weeks, 'Arthur's and his mother's relationship continued to improve. . . . Arthur was learning more movements, copying his mother's expressions, smiling at her, *and now looking into her eyes during breast-feeding.* Mother was now talking to Arthur in a loving way, telling him that he liked this and that, and rubbing his tummy, all of which had been absent earlier. *She now commented that he had begun to look at her so intently during breast-feeding that sometimes it got in the way* [by which she meant that he would stop

sucking for a while. This is 'organisation by alternation', which Bruner (1968) says typically develops between nine and thirteen weeks.] By the sixth visit Arthur seemed infatuated with his Mum, *eyes "devouring" her in their conversations....* She was copying Arthur's chatting and gurgling.... He was now enjoying bathtimes, limbs free and kicking. Earlier he had been quite stiff in the bath, eyes locked on his Mum.' [The observer has sensitively distinguished between the use of the eyes for communication and for anxious 'locking on' as described by Bick (1968).]

At twelve weeks, Arthur is coordinating eyes and mouth:

Arthur quietened as we came in and I noticed that he was holding his hands together. A moment later he drew them to his mouth and pushed them in, and began sucking the base of his thumb. As he did this he became aware of his hands visually and squinted at them. He did not persist as this seemed uncomfortable, and he stopped sucking and removed them from his mouth.

A little later in the observation, this coordination breaks down in response to an impassive face.

Mother has gone out to make tea, and Arthur shows his anxiety. The observer would like to comfort him, but feels inhibited by the demands of the role, and therefore compromises by coming physically close to Arthur but remaining impassive. 'I stood beside him and looked at him and remained motionless and expressionless, and noticed that he settled down.'

Significantly, when Mother feeds Arthur slightly after this, he reverts to the pattern of not looking at her that he had previously outgrown:

Mother gave him her left breast. *Arthur was again not looking at his mother which he had begun to do recently,* and I wondered whether this was an expression of the need for that security which only the breast could give him in the earlier weeks. He was losing himself in the experience and not connecting with Mother.... I wondered how the physical development shown today fitted in with this apparent reversal. When finished on one side Arthur stayed in position, eyes closed, semi-drugged but still attached.

I wish to stress the way in which Arthur temporarily lost the achievement of being able to look at his mother during a feed after his anxiety had been met by the observer's physical presence but seeming emotional absence. (Of course the observer was not in fact emotionally absent at all, but was trying to present a so-called neutral face.) Arthur reverted to cutting himself off visually from his mother and concentrating on the sensual experience of the feed and of the nipple, which he retained in his mouth. We might wonder how far he was identified with an impassive observer; indeed, how far he had earlier been identifying himself with an insecure mother who did things by the clock.

Fortunately, this reversal proved extremely short-lived. On the changing mat a little while later:

> Mother was keeping him informed of his experience, saying, 'You like [this] and you like [that], don't you?' Arthur was lapping it up and very involved. *His tongue came in and out of his mouth like he was trying to link this pleasurable experience with the pleasure of having the nipple in his mouth.*[2] . . . He was reaching out for his mother with his arms and hands. The smiles, fixed looks, noises, and definite first attempts at laughing . . . seemed to convey, 'I love you, Mummy.'

I find it helpful to think in terms of Arthur's preconception of an integrated object in relation to which emotion and sensuality meet up. He finds the realisation of this on the changing mat instead of at the breast. His mother felt most at ease over the changing mat: this was the setting in which he could elicit a loving response from her. When the 'meaning' he saw reflected in her eyes was a good one, his eyes and tongue came together as they did not when he met with blankness in the observer's face. The link with my post-autistic patient is obvious. Similarly, when Reid's patient Georgie (Reid 1990) had made her smile at him in a way that lit up her eyes, his own eyes lit up; he began to play with the light switch; and his mouth formed vowel shapes as he had seen hers do.

Bruner (1968) has proposed a chronology for the development of a baby's ability to integrate sucking and looking. He links this development to the maturation of the cognitive capacity to process experience on a 'dual track'. At twelve weeks, Arthur had developed 'organisation by alternation', which according to Bruner appears between nine and thirteen weeks of age. However, Mother experienced the intervals during which Arthur gazed into her eyes as interfering with the feed. Mother's sense of unease during feeds, so different from her feelings during a nappy change, might well have led her to wish that the baby should 'get it over with'. One can imagine how this might slow up the process of integration unless there is a counterbalance such as the interaction on the changing mat. The baby might well need to consolidate his experience of himself as someone good in mother's eyes before he can take responsibility for what his mouth is doing, or own a sense of agency.

In fact, the changing mat was not the only alternative to the breast that provided Arthur with the realisation of an integrated object:

> At twenty-one weeks, he was taking solids. Mother was relieved by this: she commented on the bright colour of the pureed peas she had pre-

pared for him. The observer reports: 'Whilst eating the puree . . . Arthur was waving his arms up and down between spoonfuls. He was having a real banquet . . . saliva mixed with food was being pushed in and out. . . . I saw that he was very alert to the movement of the trees as they were blown by the wind and stopped to concentrate on them for 10–15 seconds. I had seen this before but then a police or ambulance siren went off and once again he lost concentration on the food and looked up into the air as he listened to it. . . . The noise of the trains that passed nearby did not attract his attention and I presume he is now very used to that sound. I also saw him follow a rook across the garden with his eyes and head.'

Later in this observation, Mother put Arthur to the right breast with a sudden, quick movement:

She plonked him down and he took the nipple quickly, eyes closed. He opened them for a moment to look at the breast and then at Ma. [In other words, Arthur is differentiating between the breast (as part object) and Mother as whole object. According to Bruner's chronology, most babies of this age would be capable of looking and feeding at the same time: with Arthur, this achievement is not yet securely established.] *She looks at him occasionally but does not meet his gaze.* The telephone rang and she got up to answer it. As she got up, Arthur came off and was sick. He never really settled after she came back. . . . She said she preferred to feed him from the left side because it left the right hand free to do other things.

Arthur had always shown a consistent preference for the right breast; that is, for the side that did not leave Mother free to do other things. Possibly her need to feel free was related to a fear of the immediacy of the feeding relationship, as though it threatened her with being taken over.

Now that she is offering solids and the pressure of that anxiety is removed, Mother seems more confident of her ability to provide something full of life (the brightly coloured puree). This is matched by Arthur's visual relationship with the green, moving tree-tops. Like the time on the changing mat, the feed with solids provides an opportunity for realising his preconception of a lively nourishing mother to whom he relates on bodily and emotional levels at once. In this observation, his feeding is interfered with by the sound of the siren, a piercing noise which is experienced as an intrusion in the way that the comforting, background rumbling of the train is not (See Maiello, Chapter 10). It is interesting to see Arthur attempting to carry over the linking of mouth and eyes, established on the changing mat and over solids in the garden, to the breast when he looks first at the breast itself and then at his mother, who does not, however, return his gaze.

The next observation I will quote from shows the baby responding by a disjunction of eyes and mouth and by psychosomatic reactions when the mother cannot acknowledge the traumatic nature of a separation.

BABY JENNY: THE SPLITTING OF EYES AND MOUTH FOLLOWING AN UNACKNOWLEDGED TRAUMA

This little girl, also a first child, had had a close, idyllic relationship with her mother for the first months. Eye contact featured prominently from early on, and mother and baby were extremely responsive to each other. The observer became increasingly uncomfortable when it became clear that mother intended to accompany her husband on an exciting holiday. Mother obviously felt that this was essential to her marriage. The point I wish to stress is that she *dealt with the conflict by pretending that it did not exist.*

The two-week separation took place when Jenny was five months old. She was left in the care of a temporary nanny. When the observer called during the parents' absence, she learned from the nanny that:

'Jenny had developed a high temperature for two days immediately after her parents' departure. Her GP found no cause. A patch of eczema had appeared on her right cheek and her sleeping increased, now accounting for sixteen hours in twenty-four.' Jenny had previously been alert and wakeful in the day, and this was completely unlike her. The nanny emphasised how well Jenny had been eating and sleeping, that she was 'just great', but added, 'She just stares and stares.' When Jenny was brought into the room, she stared, expressionless, at the observer to whom she did not give her usual smile. There was another child present, at whom Jenny stared anxiously with occasional smiles. After a time, the nanny sat Jenny in her high chair and prepared to feed her. 'As Jenny started to feed she turned to me, stared, and after a few seconds smiled. This pattern continued for the whole feed, with Jenny looking and staring at me, and smiling, and then turning for a few seconds to look at the nanny [who was feeding her], and then back to me for long stretches. I stared back, occasionally smiling or just staring too. Jenny polished off her solids and continued staring, half smiling, at me. The nanny lifted up her coffee to drink and Jenny looked at her, staring, as though to fathom her out, and then returned to stare at me . . .' The nanny seemed disconcerted, and stimulated Jenny by jiggling her and smiling at her; Jenny then did respond by smiling back.

Jenny's reaction to the separation is largely somatic: she develops eczema and seems to be using sleep as a means of withdrawal. Although her eating is 'ever so good', the quality of her stare disconcerts both the nanny and the observer. It seems to be saying, in a way that her actions do not: 'You are not someone I want or even recognise.' Apart from the obvious reasons for this – after all, through no fault of hers, the nanny was indeed the wrong person – one might relate the stare of non-recognition to mother's inability to acknowledge either her own mixed feelings about the separation or its likely effect on the little girl. The mother may well be felt to be unresponsive because she is occupied by another baby: Jenny accords the same alternation of stares and smiles to the observer and to the other child. Jenny's response recalls the way in which Arthur went blank after he met with an expressionless observer: he went on to retreat from the achievement of looking at his mother during a breast-feed. Similarly, Jenny divides up her mouth and her eyes between the observer, whom she looks at for long stretches, and the nanny, who feeds her but whom she hardly looks at.

Shortly after her parents' return, Jenny was introduced to a different nanny, who was to look after her regularly when her mother returned to work. This was to begin in a few days; after a week, the whole family were to leave for a skiing holiday during which Jenny was to be in a crèche.

> Jenny became distressed during the visit, and turned towards Mother appealingly. She remained straight-backed, refusing to intervene, stating that the nanny had to learn how to cope.

This does not do justice to the atmosphere of the whole visit: the observer was in no doubt that Mother was in fact feeling very torn, and was herself finding it hard to 'learn how to cope'. The next observation I will quote from occurred after a two-week break, when Jenny was twenty-eight weeks old.

> In spite of the interruption, 'Jenny looked well and smiled in response to my hello, kicking her legs in pleasure.' Mother explained that she had been in hospital, following what appeared to be a violent allergic reaction to egg. She had been acutely distressed and had had trouble breathing. [A year and a half later, Mother told the observer that hospital tests had conclusively established that Jenny was not allergic to eggs. No medical explanation had been suggested for her sudden dramatic illness.] When Mother left the room to prepare lunch, Jenny grew restless and grizzled, but responded for quite some time by playing with the toys the observer gave her. Then, as 'I was sitting quietly on the floor alongside her. . . . Jenny, using her left hand, grabbed the side bar of the play gym and pulled herself half onto her left side, then she turned and fixed her gaze on me for five or ten seconds before turning away again, her expression still and impassive. She again turned back to me, stared and after a few seconds turned her back to me. She repeated this about five times and I wondered if she was making me go and re-appear. . . . Mother came into the room and I was struck that

Jenny in no way acknowledged the sound of her approaching footsteps and voice. I felt uncomfortable and tried to locate an external reason for Jenny's lack of response. . . .

As Mother bent to pick Jenny up, her eyes lighted on her food and her hands flapped with excitement and anticipation. Jenny greeted each spoonful with a satisfied "hmmmm!", singing as she ate. She opened her mouth like a hungry bird waiting for the next morsel. Halfway down the jar Jenny shut her eyes, turned her head from side to side and refused any more. . . . Mother then gave Jenny some mashed banana and, again, Jenny had five or six spoonful, then stopped and grizzled. Mother responded, "You've had enough, then?" *During the whole of the feed Jenny's eyes were fixed to the left of Mother's head as she waited for each spoonful and she didn't look at Mother once.* Mother was saying that Jenny had been "great" in the crèche from nine till five, and what a relief that had been: "My friend's baby, who is the same age, howls if her mum leaves the room; I couldn't bear that."

A little later, Jenny began to grizzle, and Mother said that she was tired, but not yet ready to sleep. She reached out for a little monkey "that Jenny loves" and shook it in front of Jenny, which made its long arms flap from side to side. Jenny's breathing became quicker, almost panting, her eyes wide. She reached out towards it, but Mother kept on shaking it. Suddenly Jenny let out an agonised cry, had a sharp intake of breath which she held for a few seconds before emitting a huge sobbing sound, her face a purple red with the intensity of her emotion. I was startled, wondering if the monkey had hit Jenny. Mother looked taken aback, even shocked, and she immediately gathered up a disintegrating Jenny and began saying, "Sorry, Jenny", and to me, "I didn't think she wanted it so much." As Jenny quietened she reached out and touched the monkey's face. . . .

Jenny became restless and seemed tired. Mother was semi-reclining on the sofa with Jenny lying on her. . . . Jenny began to push hard against Mother until she started moving off. "Jenny, no," said Mother, and pulled her back. . . . Mother was talking to Jenny and saying "shh . . .", but Jenny was turning her head from left to right *as though avoiding Mother's face* and again began to push against Mother and slide down her body.

Mother became exasperated by Jenny's avoidance of eye contact, and she picked her up, holding her aloft, almost forcing Jenny to fix on her, which Jenny did for a few seconds and smiled. Mother placed Jenny on her chest again and this time Jenny let her head fall on her mother's chest, sucked her thumb and her eyelids grew heavy. She grew a little restless, then suddenly opened her eyes and fixed on me for ten seconds quite expressionless. She half reached out towards me, then stopped and began sucking her thumb and drifted to sleep.'

I wish to emphasise only a few points of this very moving observation. Jenny has managed to retain at least something of a good relationship with her mother by taking refuge in the sensual enjoyment of feeding, but the split between eye and mouth has carried over from the previous observation. (This split is not complete: she rejects food by turning her head from side to side, a similar movement to that in the game of making the observer disappear and in her later avoidance of her mother's face.) Possibly strengthened by the sense of mastery she gained in the game with the observer, possibly simply overcome by the intensity of her feeling which is such as to make the observer think she had been physically hurt, she stops being 'good' in the incident with the monkey. Mother is now shaken and responsive, and feels pain when her baby wriggles away and avoids her face instead of welcoming the absence of demands. With this re-establishment of communication, Jenny is able to snuggle down against her mother and go to sleep *with her thumb in her mouth*. She takes a last step towards integrating the experience of mother's absence by reaching out towards the observer with a blank stare, before sleep overcomes her. I feel that the presence of an observer who could tolerate the pain of the blank stare during mother's absence and understand the reason for it must have been of great help to her.

I will now quote briefly from an observation that shows even more clearly how the communication and containment of feeling can heal a disjunction between eyes and mouth. In this case, it is the observer who feels pain for most of the visit.[3]

BABY JULIET: FOOD AS A SUBSTITUTE FOR MEANING

This sixteen-week-old baby girl was the second child in her family, where her father was said to be 'the better mother'. At the beginning of the observation:

> Mother is on her way out to work, looking reluctant to go. Father's parents are there, so is Juliet's brother: there is a general feeling of too many people in the house. Father hands Juliet to the observer while he makes tea: Juliet had not reacted adversely when she first saw the observer, but now 'Juliet looked at me stunned for a few seconds, and then her face crumpled into misery and a strong forlorn wail came forth.' The observer tried to calm her, but without success. Father reappeared suddenly, whisked Juliet away and asked her what the matter was, but she continued to wail miserably whenever she saw the observer's face. 'It seemed as if each time she looked at me and registered that it was not a familiar face, she became very unhappy and cried her heart out. I felt rather miserable too, and wanted to sit out of her line of vision. . . . Father spoke quietly and calmly and was

sympathetic to her misery. He would ask her what was wrong and try to think what was the cause. He mentioned that she has had some solids over the past few weeks, thinking it could be wind, and I was shown the apple-pear baby jar and the amount which she takes for lunch. . . . He cooed at her, rocking her in his arms. It did not seem that anything relieved her more than very momentarily. At one point he heard her expel something into her nappy and he said, "Ahah! That's what's been bothering you!" But she soon picked up again and cried on. I put it to Father that Juliet might be upset because of her mother's absence, and he said without conviction that it was possible . . .'

The observation goes on, with Father trying everything he can think of and finally offering Juliet the bottle.

She refuses it at first, but 'with his persevering, she took the bottle which seemed to be the only time she was not crying. As she became more settled and sucked well from the bottle, Father spoke very quietly and soothingly to her. . . . Juliet and her father held each other in their gaze for quite a time. When he retracted the bottle, Juliet stayed quiet for a few minutes until she was sat up and caught sight of me which seemed to start her crying pitifully. He laid her back in his arms and gave her the bottle again which she took more readily.' Father then discusses times of visits with the observer: these will have to be moved to accommodate Mother's schedule. Then he takes the bottle from Juliet's mouth, and checks how much she has had: he comments that she was having a lot today, this was her third bottle. Juliet starts to cry again persistently and the observer feels dismayed. Father returns the bottle to her and wonders whom she will take after, whether she will have a temper. He makes faces to interest her, then apologises to the observer for Juliet's behaviour, saying to Juliet that the observer might be disappointed to see her like this when she was usually so good. 'I replied that, on the contrary, I was sorry to see that she was having a tough time today but it was a hectic time for everyone and I could see she got fed up sometimes.'

Father, thinking she might be tired, tries to settle Juliet in her room. She relaxes briefly, but when he tries to interest her in a favourite toy:

'she intently stared at her father. Then she started to cry loudly again.' Back in the kitchen, 'while she continued to cry, he walked her around slowly, gently rocking her and soothing her with his quiet voice. He said to her that he guessed that life was not so good for her right now. Slowly, very slowly, she calmed down with her father staring fixedly into her face, rhythmically passing his hand over her brow and head, while gently rocking her in his arms. She stopped crying and emitted instead deep, soulful sighs for quite a time.'

I have quoted from this observation because it so clearly illustrates the transformatory power of emotional containment. Throughout the visit, it was the observer who suffered the pain of being the wrong person, the one who made Juliet cry. Father dismissed the observer's early suggestion that Juliet might be missing her mother, but he was able to pick up on her comment towards the end that Juliet might be finding life hard just now. The contrast brings out the difference between an accurate explanation that does not address the pain in the situation it describes, and a transforming intervention that grows out of the struggle with this pain.

It is clear that the bottle is not really what Juliet wants, but like Jenny she takes refuge in the sensual gratification. As she calms down, and Father is relieved, they look at each other for a long time: at this moment eye and mouth can come together. The sight of the observer's face reminds her of her distress, however, and one feels that she turns more readily to the bottle to escape it. She persists however in letting Father know that there is still something wrong, and at the end he is able to comfort her without recourse to food. One can only speculate on how many extra bottles she might have had otherwise, and on what her relationship to food might have become had this pattern persisted.

CONCLUSION

In *Learning from Experience*, Bion suggests: 'It is likely from clinical evidence of the infant's need for material and psychological support that no distinction between material and psychological can be made by the infant. In analysis, however, it is possible to deduce whether the deficiency was one of physical or psychical quality' (Bion 1962: 29). He probably had in mind babies younger than the three I have been discussing, each of whom in addition had enjoyed a basically good relationship with its mother. While these observations enable us to distinguish between the material and psychological components of what is provided for the infant I think that they also show the babies themselves making this distinction very clearly. The way in which Arthur tried to transfer his visual relationship with his mother from changing mat or solids to breast seems to me strong evidence for a preconception of a mother with distinct but interrelated mental and material qualities; what I have called an integrated object, the experience of which of course will serve to promote integration.

Bion writes also of the way in which the infant's inability to tolerate the mother's emotional support may lead to an insatiable demand for creature comforts which in the end never satisfy. The infants in these three observations did not suffer greatly from this difficulty, but one can see, particularly with Juliet, how sensuality could hypertrophy in the absence of emotional understanding. A complication that is often encountered can arise when the caregiver does not feel confident of having anything to offer emotionally, and turns to the breast or bottle as a panacea. This was true to a certain extent of Juliet's father.

These observations illustrate temporary disruptions in the integration of mind and body that can occur when emotional contact between baby and caregiver is interfered with. They also show how this harmony can be restored when the caregiver (or the observer!) is open to the communication of feeling. The implications are obvious for autistic states, where Frances Tustin has emphasised the importance of a 'mental uterus' in which the baby is held (Tustin 1980) as well as for eating disorders and other psychosomatic problems. This line of thought may also be relevant to patients who cannot tolerate the couch because of an imperative need for eye contact (see Searles 1963, on the importance of the therapist's face). If we think in terms of the baby's preconception of an integrated and integrating object, then a defective sense of agency or hypertrophied sensuality can be seen as a retreat from the perceived implications of eye contact rather than as a failure to develop.

ACKNOWLEDGEMENTS

I am grateful to the observers, unnamed for discretion's sake, for allowing me to quote material from their infant observations.

I wish to express my thanks to the *British Journal of Psychotherapy* for allowing me to make use of quotations from the infant observation and my commentary on it which appeared there as part of the Clinical Commentary section [*British Journal of Psychotherapy 9*: 476, 1993 (Rhode 1993)].

I am grateful to A.P. Watts for permission to reprint the lines from 'Drinking Song' by W.B. Yeats. Reprinted with the permission of Simon & Schuster from *The Collected Works of W. B. Yeats, Volume I: The Poems*, revised edited by Richard J. Finneran (New York: Macmillan, 1989).

NOTES

1 When these ideas were first presented in my paper read to the Infant Observation Conference, the point was made repeatedly in discussion that the eye is itself a physical structure, so that the correspondence between eye contact and meaning on the one hand, and mouth contact and sensation on the other can be a very rough one at best. Anne Alvarez pointed out that an infant can have a complete, object-related experience at the breast with its eyes closed. I agree completely with this: the equivalence I am proposing is no more than schematic, and the eye implies 'the eye with the mind behind it' (Judith Jackson). The interplay between eye and mouth will undoubtedly evolve in the move between primary and introjective identification (cf. Wright's (1991) treatment of the development of symbolic space).

2 The tongue here is used in exploratory mode, rather than as a source of self-

generated sensation (Tustin 1981). For a discussion of the importance of the tongue, see Bonnard (1960)

3 The infant observation summarised here was published in the *British Journal of Psychotherapy* (1993) 9: 476 ff. The material was discussed by three psychotherapists of differing orientations as part of a Clinical Commentary (Rhode 1993).

REFERENCES

Alvarez, A. (1992) *Live Company*, London and New York: Tavistock/Routledge.

Bick, E. (1968) 'The experience of the skin in early object relations', *International Journal of Psycho-Analysis*, 49: 484–486.

Bion, W. R. (1950) 'The imaginary twin', in *Second Thoughts: Selected Papers on Psycho-Analysis*, London: Heinemann (1967; reprinted in paperback: Maresfield Reprints, London: Karnac Books, 1984).

Bion, W. R. (1962) *Learning from Experience*, London: Heinemann (reprinted in paperback: Maresfield Reprints, London: Karnac Books, 1984).

Bonnard, A. (1960) 'The primal significance of the tongue', *International Journal of Psycho-Analysis*, 41: 301–307.

Bruner, J. S. (1968) *Processes of Cognitive Growth: Infancy*, Worcester, MA.: Clark University Press.

Freud, S. (1923). 'The ego and the id', *Standard Edition* 19: 3–66. London: Hogarth (1966).

Haag, G. (1984) 'Autisme infantile précoce et phénomènes autistiques. Réflexions psychanalytiques', *Psychiatrie de l'enfant*, 27: 293–354.

Haag, G. (1991) 'Contribution à la compréhension des identifications en jeu dans le moi corporel', paper read at the Congress of the International Psychoanalytical Association, Buenos Aires.

Haag, G. (1992) 'Fear of fusion and projective identification in autistic children', *Psychoanalytic Inquiry*, 13: 63–83. A modified version of this paper is included in M. Rustin, H. Dubinsky, A. Dubinsky and M. Rhode (eds) *Psychotic States in Children and Adolescents*, in press.

Klein, M. (1952) 'On observing the behaviour of young infants', in *Envy and Gratitude and Other Works: The Writings of Melanie Klein*, Vol. III, London: Hogarth and the Institute of Psycho-Analysis (1975).

Klein, S. (1965) 'Notes on a case of ulcerative colitis', *International Journal of Psycho-Analysis*, 46: 342–351.

Klein, S. (1980) 'Autistic phenomena in neurotic patients', *International Journal of Psycho-Analysis*, 61: 395–402.

Klein, S. (1984) 'Delinquent perversion: problems of assimilation: a clinical study', *International Journal of Psycho-Analysis*, 65: 307–314.

McDougall, J. (1989) *Theatres of the Body*, London: Free Association Books.

Meltzer, D. (1986) *Studies in Extended Metapsychology*. Strath Tay, Perthshire: Clunie Press.

Meltzer, D., Bremner, J., Hoxter, S., Weddell, D. and Wittenberg, I. (1975) *Explorations in Autism*, Strath Tay, Perthshire: Clunie Press.

Meltzoff, A. and Barton, R. (1979) 'Intermodal matching by human neonates', *Nature*, 282: 403–404.

Negri, R. (1994) *The Newborn in the Intensive Care Unit: A Neuropsychoanalytic Prevention Model*, London: Clunie Press/Karnac Books.

Pines, M. (1987) 'Mirroring and child development: psychodynamic and psychological interpretations', in K. Yardley and T. Honess (eds) *Self and Identity: Psychoanalytical Perspectives*, Chichester: Wiley.

Pines, M. (1993) Unpublished paper read to the Parent-Infant Clinic, London.

Reid, S. (1990) 'The importance of beauty in the psychoanalytic experience', *Journal of Child Psychotherapy*, 16: 29–52.

Rhode, M. (1993) Contribution to 'Clinical Commentary', *British Journal of Psychotherapy*, 9: 483–485.

Ryz, P. (1993) 'Obsessionality, communication and mis-communication', *Journal of Child Psychotherapy*, 19: 47–62.

Searles, H. F. (1963) 'The place of neutral therapist responses in psychotherapy with the schizophrenic patient', in *Collected Papers on Schizophrenia and Related Subjects*, London: Hogarth (1965; reprinted in paperback, London: Karnac Books, 1986).

Spitz, R. A. (1955) 'The primal cavity', *The Psychoanalytic Study of the Child*, 10: 215–240.

Stern, D. (1985) *The Interpersonal World of the Infant*, New York: Basic Books.

Tustin, F. (1980) 'Psychological birth and psychological catastrophe', in J. S. Grotstein (ed.) *Do I Dare Disturb the Universe?* Beverly Hills: Caesura Press, 1981 (reprinted in paperback, Maresfield Reprints, London: Karnac Books, 1983; also in F. Tustin 1981).

Tustin, F. (1981) *Autistic States in Children*, London: Routledge, 2nd revised edition, 1992.

Tustin, F. (1994) 'The perpetuation of an error', *Journal of Child Psychotherapy*, 20: 3–23.

Winnicott, D. W. (1967) 'Mirror-role of mother and family in child development', in *Playing and Reality*, London: Tavistock Publications (1971; reprinted in paperback, London: Routledge, 1991).

Wright, K. (1991) *Vision and Separation between Mother and Baby*, London: Free Association Books.

Yeats, W. B. (1910) 'A Drinking Song', in W. B. Yeats: *Collected Poems*, London: Macmillan, 1963.

Chapter 10

Interplay

Sound-aspects in mother–infant observation

Suzanne Maiello

INTRODUCTION

Infant observation has proved to be not only a fundamental tool of students' training, but has often become both the source and the testing-ground of ideas and theoretical hypotheses about the earliest stages of mental life.

There are two reasons for giving special attention to sound-aspects in infant observation material, and in particular to vocal interaction between mother and infant. First, it seems important to try to understand more about the meaning of auditory experiences for the infant, and search for evidence for the hypothesis of the existence of pre-natal sound-memories connected in particular with the mother's voice (Maiello 1995). Second, the increase of the observers' awareness and sensitivity to sound- and vocal aspects of the mother–infant interplay, which often contain important elements of meaning, will widen and deepen their comprehension of the global situation.

It is a fact that we live in a more and more visually oriented world and that our civilisation tends to neglect the differentiating capacity of hearing, to the detriment of a more global perception of things. The ancient Chinese used to refer to the hearing faculty which led to enlightenment and knowledge as the 'light of the ears'.

Sound seems to precede visual manifestation both in cultural and individual development. The ethno-musicologist M. Schneider (1992: 13) asserts that in almost all cultures the creative source of the world is a sound, either a cry or a crash of thunder or a song, which then generates light and clarity. Before acquiring shapes and faces, the gods were rhythms and melodies. 'Music is located between the obscurity of unconscious life and the clarity of mental representations' (Schneider 1992: 20).

The infant's first act at the moment of birth is a cry. It is the moment of transition from obscurity to light. An Italian expression for 'being born' is *'venire alla luce'*, coming to light. But whilst the child's first sound-production coincides with its coming to light, its sound-perception has already a long history up to that moment.

The results of neurophysiological research (Tomatis 1987; Prechtl 1989) show that the hearing capacity of the human foetus is completely developed by the age of four months of intra-uterine life. By that time, the foetus perceives the medium and high sound frequency range corresponding to the mother's voice. The low frequency range corresponding to the sounds produced by the maternal organism (the heart-beat, the cadence of breathing and the digestional noises), are perceived at an even earlier stage. Furthermore, Piontelli's observational study (1992: 23) gives striking evidence of the consistency of children's behaviour before and after birth. This in turn confirms findings (Tomatis 1987: 55) which show that the mother's voice is not only heard by the unborn child, but its sound and timbre, its rhythmical and musical qualities, become the actual base for its future linguistic code.

In psychoanalytical terms, this means that the child must be capable, already before being born, of some form of introjection. Isaacs (1952: 105) describes the complex process of development of phantasy from the concrete experience of the infant's somatic sensations, with their prevalent quality of 'me-ness', to its gradual integration with visual elements. The increase of the latter brings about the differentiation of inner from outer world and the possibility of the introjection of images, as well as the repression of the more concrete elements of perception and phantasy. No specific mention is made by Isaacs of auditory experiences and of the introjection of sound-elements. Today, the results of recent research suggest on the one hand the idea that some form of introjection occurs already during pre-natal life, and on the other that the introjected elements have at least partly sound-qualities deriving from the child's perception of the mother's voice. Furthermore, the alternation of the sound of her voice and her silence may give the unborn child a very first experience of both presence and absence, and thus become the basis for the constitution of a pre-natal proto-object, which I tentatively called 'sound-object' (Maiello 1995: 28). Extending Isaacs's formulation to pre-natal life, it might be suggested that auditory phantasies could be located somewhere half-way between the primary concrete somatic experiences present already before birth, and the visual representations which are still latent in the obscurity of the womb and begin to develop only after the child has 'come to light'. Pre-natal auditory experiences and memories might already entail some rudimentary differentiation between 'me' and 'not-me'. They might be located somewhere between material reality and representation. In fact, the area of sounds and vocality can be said to be not yet symbolic, but at the very root of symbolisation. The voice does not represent feelings, but is itself the representative of emotional states. Sounds emerge from memory through evocation, and their level of expression corresponds to the area of 'song-and-dance' (Meltzer *et al.* 1986: 185), in which container/ contained are not yet distinct, but on the verge of differentiation. 'Lalling and babbling' (Meltzer *et al.* 1986: 185) may be seen to occur on the threshold between vocal music and verbal communication.

Vocal interplay between mother and child is normally intensely present from birth, and material from infant observations may give a deeper insight into this area and bring about better understanding of the meaning of the communication at sound-level.

THE MOTHER'S VOICE

There is a very particular way in which adults talk to babies, and any listener would be able to make out that this kind of talk is addressed to a baby or maybe to a pet, even if he only overheard the voice without seeing the scene. Adults seem to find spontaneously the tone and quality of voice to which a baby's ear is attuned, and which therefore is able to elicit a reaction. T. B. Brazelton (1973: 23) states that the best animate auditory stimulus for the infant is continuous, soft and high-pitched speech. In fact, when turning to an infant, the adult's voice is naturally at a higher pitch than in conversation with other adults or older children. Also, it is more melodious and more rhythmical. It has a singing and swaying quality, a rising or falling tonality, according to its emotional function which may be either stimulating or soothing. The semantic meaning of words is less important than their sound- and rhythm-value. Such rhythmic and musical language is present for instance in nursery rhymes: 'Hush-a-bye baby on the tree top', or 'Humpty Dumpty sat on a wall'.

A first example of material drawn from an infant observation shows the importance of the mother's tone of voice as carrier of an emotional message.

> Diana is three weeks old on the observer's first visit. While holding the baby against her chest for the observer to see her, the mother gives an account of her difficult delivery. She speaks in a calm and soft voice. It sounds as if she were re-evoking with her baby the hard time they both had. She says how sorry she is for having been unable to control herself and for screaming with pain during the long labour. Diana starts having a hiccup while her mother talks, but does not seem to be bothered too much by it. The mother feels that it is better to wait for the hiccup to stop before laying her down, because she knows that otherwise the baby will cry. She then turns her daughter around and talks to her tenderly. The hiccup stops soon, and the mother tells Diana in a lulling and swinging tone that she will now put her to sleep. 'Ora andiamo a nanna,' she says.

At this point, the limits of a written text become evident. In fact, it is often difficult and sometimes impossible to reproduce the vocal timbre and musical qualities of oral language in writing. But whenever there is an opportunity for oral exchange, such as in infant observation seminars or clinical supervision, re-evoking the sound-quality of vocal communications often becomes a very important element for a fuller understanding of the material.

The observation of Diana and her mother continues:

> The mother lays the baby in the cot and gives her the dummy. Diana sucks vigorously, but soon loses it and starts whimpering. The mother comes back from the kitchen and puts the dummy back into the baby's mouth, while talking to her softly and saying that she knows Diana will fall asleep soon. She loses the dummy a second time and whimpers again. The noises of dish washing come over from the kitchen, together with the sound of mother's voice that hums a song. The baby stops complaining and lies alert. She visibly listens and soon quiets down. Her mouth makes sucking movements, which gradually become slower. Her eyes close, and she falls asleep.

In this example, the mother's voice in the baby's ears seemed to have been a sufficient presence for her to hold on to and go to sleep without the dummy filling her mouth. The mother's capacity to integrate frustrating and painful memories (her regretful feelings about having screamed during delivery) allowed her also to bear the baby's hiccup and whimpering without anxiety, and later for Diana to have the experience that the potentially persecutory loss of the dummy and the consequent anxiety expressed by her whimpering were safely contained and soothed by mother's singing voice.

Another example may show how, on the contrary, a mother's fear of deep emotional involvement as well as denied persecutory anxieties find expression in the tone of her voice, depriving it of its communication-stimulating musical quality.

During the interview before birth, the observer was struck both by the mother's absence of imagination of the baby that was to be born, and by her intense fear of delivery. On the observer's first visit, Emilio was two weeks old.

> The mother is relieved that he is such a good baby and never cries. When she puts him to the breast, he has difficulty in grasping the nipple and loses it many times before settling down and sucking. As soon as he drinks regularly, the mother turns to the observer to tell her about her dramatic delivery. Her eyes and hands are hardly ever in contact with the child. At one point, some milk goes down the wrong way. The baby's face turns red, he struggles and coughs. The mother comments

in a flat, matter-of-fact tone of voice: 'You're choking', but does nothing to help Emilio to recover.

Just like her eyes, hands and nipple, this mother's voice did not have any inflection that could have created an emotional link with her baby. Emilio had learnt very quickly not to reach out, not to cry and not to look, and to be what the mother called a good baby. Later, he was to become a tense, hyperactive and bossy child, with a muscular shell and very early motor development. When he was about ten months old, he used to beat his chest with both fists like a gorilla and to scream as loudly as he could, in a state of mind which felt to the observer to be a very painful and uncontainable mixture of excitement and despair. Emilio's language development too was precocious. He learned early to pronounce correctly even difficult words, but had done very little lalling and babbling 'baby-talk'.

THE BABY'S VOICE

Little thought has been given so far to the importance and meaning of one particular capacity that the infant acquires at the moment of birth: the use of its voice, and in general the production of sounds. At the visual level, the unborn child is unseen and unseeing. At the auditory level, a kind of dialogue is already going on: the child hears the mother's voice, although its response has still to find other channels of expression, such as motor activity or changes in the rhythm of heart-beat. Birth brings about the possibility for actual one-to-one vocal exchange.

The following example will show how a baby discovers its yet unknown capacity to use its voice for communication.

> Giulia is eight weeks old. She has just had her breast-feed and lies in her infant seat, which rocks softly as she moves her arms and legs. Her mother is leaning over her and talks to her tenderly. Giulia responds with bright smiles, and the rhythm of her motor activity increases. Something very intense seems to seek expression from inside. Her eyes are in her mother's eyes. She smiles again and moves her mouth and tongue until she produces a gurgling little sound. The thrusting movements of her arms and legs increase further. Her mother continues to talk to her in a soft tone, with occasional silences, as if she wanted to give the baby a chance to reply. The expression on Giulia's face is intensely communicative. She opens her mouth wider, moves her tongue again in all directions and at last emits a loud, high, joyful-sounding little cry. Immediately, her arm and leg movements stop, and the previously rocking relaxing chair stands still. For a moment, her eyes leave her mother's face and seem vaguely searching. The expression on her face is of wonder and surprise. She is motionless, but alert, her attention

somehow inward-bound, as if she were still listening to the echo of the extraordinary unknown sound that has come out of her.

This observation shows both the intense emotional and communicative significance of vocal interaction and the overwhelmingly strong motivation of the baby to learn to use its voice and to articulate sounds that are precursors of verbal communication. The sounds produced by the baby are elicited by the adult's vocal expressions and vice versa, in an ongoing reciprocal stimulation. But it could be suggested as well that the evident intensity of the baby's wish for vocal communication might stem also from its pre-natal auditory experience of the mother's voice. Even though its sound, filtered through the amniotic liquid, is not identical with the voice the child hears after birth, there seem to be sufficient melodious and rhythmical elements to characterise it unmistakably. Could meeting the mother's voice again after birth be said to be the realisation of what has been internalised as a sound-object during pre-natal life? And vocalisation the expression of this internalised sound-object?

Another question concerns the extension to the father and other persons of this passionate dialogue. Could it in part be due to the baby's already introjected capacity to sense the musical essence of loving attention in other than the mother's voice? Listening to Giulia, it is interesting to note the slight differences in the dialogues she had with her mother and with her father. With him, her attention was somehow more focused and her talk more articulate, while when communicating with her mother, her passion seemed at times to have a quietly fulfilled flavour, with her mouth and tongue and lips producing a mixture of sucking and sound-articulating movements.

INTROJECTION OF PRE-NATAL AND EARLY POST-NATAL AUDITORY EXPERIENCES

Tomatis (1987: 37–42) writes about an observation made in his clinical practice with a child who had been adopted shortly after birth by a Spanish-speaking South American family. The child was emotionally withdrawn, and his speech was flat and unexpressive. He came to life again and started babbling with an unmistakably Portuguese intonation when he heard Port-uguese spoken. The author concluded that the child must have had a Brazilian mother.

Another example that seems to give evidence of some form of pre-natal experience comes from an adolescent who was born and raised in Italy by his Italian father and his bilingual Italian and German mother. The family language had always been Italian. During his studies, he took a German language course. As he heard the teacher speak for the first time, he was overwhelmed by the most intense emotion at the sound of this foreign language. He found out later that his mother had been back to Germany for a few weeks during the second half of pregnancy and had obviously spoken German during her stay.

The above examples seem to testify to some form of pre-natal auditory memory. The observation material that follows gives evidence of early post-natal internalisation of the mother's voice.

> Giovanni is two months old. He smiles and vocalises a lot. When his mother puts him to sleep, she often plays singing games with him, and the baby responds with joyful sounds, moving his arms and legs. When his response becomes less active, the mother turns him to one side, pulls the bedsheet up to cover him and pushes his cot to and fro while singing a lullaby in a low and tender voice. The baby emits soft humming sounds as the mother sings. His eyes gradually close and he falls asleep. Four months later, Giovanni has been weaned, and his mother has gone back to work. During the day, he is looked after by his aunt. When she puts him down to sleep in the pram, the baby holds tightly on to the bedsheet with one hand, the other hand lightly strokes his face, and his voice produces the same soft continuous sounds with which he used to accompany his mother's lullabies. He goes on humming until his breath slows down, his arms slide along his body and his eyes close.

He seems to have learnt to sing himself to sleep even without his mother.

When a baby is born and becomes capable of using its voice, the obvious function is that of drawing the attention of the baby's surroundings to its needs. Later, when the child starts speaking, we recognise the power acquired over external objects by the capacity to give them names. It might be suggested that a similar power is acquired by the baby as soon as it has a voice of its own. In phantasy, the baby can get hold of and reproduce precisely that part of the pre-natal world that escaped its control during the first mute part of its life, namely, the mother's voice. Giovanni's singing was not imitative. He was capable of recreating a good and pro-tecting sound-object when his mother was absent.

SOUND AND MEANING

Pre-natal sound-perception can be evaluated and described with fair pre-cision. However, what the unborn child's experience is when it hears the mother's voice and listens to her talk, remains an open question. Are the sounds it perceives 'only' melody and rhythm, or is there already some rudimentary need and ability to grasp emotional meaning in the sounds it hears? The foetus shows clearly that it distinguishes vocal presence from vocal absence (Tomatis 1987: 61). Is it possible that it is also able to sense a difference between 'good' and 'bad' sounds, a 'good' and a 'bad' voice? Between accepting and refusing vocal messages? In other words, can we imagine some sort of pre-natal precursor of a differentiating capacity at sound level?

The following example does not answer this question, but shows that sounds are clearly connected with meanings in mother–infant interaction.

The observer's first visit to the newborn baby's family left her with a wonderful feeling of warmth and harmony, which was to last for the first weeks of Beatrice's life. The mother was in deep contact with the baby; she talked softly and continuously with her and followed and interpreted every one of her movements and expressions. She gave her long and pleasurable massages, to which the infant abandoned herself with relish. One day, while breast-feeding her, she commented on her milk as an aphrodisiac. 'We love it, don't we, Bea?' (pronounced 'Bear'.) She always used the plural form 'we' until Beatrice was four months old.

The baby had started giving the first signs of discomfort during massages at about two months of age. Ecstatic beatitude and abandonment alternated with moments when she frowned and seemed to try to withdraw from her mother's caressing hands. It was quite obvious that the mother's fusional phantasies began to be an obstacle to the baby's incipient need for separation and differentiation. Beatrice now began to cry as soon as her mother started changing her, and sometimes went on in a crescendo until she screamed in despair. But the mother did not take much notice of her child's state of mind and would not modify the pattern of intense physical contact and control over her.

At four months of age, Beatrice's crying began to sound less desperate and developed a more angry and aggressive quality instead. She produced guttural sounds in her throat, which her mother compared to the roaring of a lion. It was at that point that she started calling her daughter BIA (pronounced 'Bee-ar'). Weaning occurred abruptly at the age of five months. The mother had fallen ill with a violent attack of flu, and her milk had gone. She rationalised the loss by saying that the first teeth would be growing soon anyway and that she had been told they could hurt and damage mothers' nipples. From that time, she would call her daughter BIKI (pronounced 'Beekee') every time she referred to such unpleasant things as the child's aggressive teeth or the persistant anal and vaginal irritation which Beatrice suffered from the moment of weaning.

For this mother, the good things were represented by softness, fusion and harmony. Separation, differentiation and individuality were felt to be hard and bad. In this example, the split between the idealised good and the persecutory bad object went right through and down into the sound-quality of words. Soft vowels and consonants were felt to be good, pleasurable and gratifying. BEA (Bear) was mother's beloved massage baby. When Beatrice began needing some more distance from her mother and started crying and screaming in protest, she became BIA (Bee-ar), and later, in connection with the idea of her teeth, BIKI (Beekee). The acute vowels and hard consonants seem to have been felt to be bad, penetrating, hurting and irritating objects and expressed the mother's anger and refusal of her daughter's changing needs. The shrill sounds of the baby's voice, whose message was not acceptable to her mother, were translated by her into the new versions of her name and put back into the child unheard and not understood.

LOSS OF PRE-NATAL SOUND-MEMORIES

Piontelli's observations of infantile amnesia of pre-natal life (1993: 13), which she reported for children from the age of about 4, found confirmation in the material of young child observations, especially as far as the sound-aspect of pre-natal or early post-natal experience is concerned. The following material may witness both the presence and loss of such early memories.

Irina was a little girl of almost 4. She had had quite a difficult time lately. After several attempts to send her to nursery school, her parents had decided to keep her at home for another year. The mother had some difficulties in letting this second and last child go, and for Irina herself it was not easy to leave her home, and especially the large armchair where she used to cuddle up whenever she encountered frustrations she could not bear. On the other hand, she longed intensely to be a schoolgirl like her 8-year-old sister. The observation material shows Irina's difficult transition from babyhood to childhood.

The children are on the square in front of the house. Irina rides her little tricycle. She tries to catch up with the group of older children who swiftly pass by on their bicycles, shouting something to her that she does not seem to understand. They disappear again around the corner. Irina pedals on a little and then gets off her bicycle. She frowns, hits the saddle with her hand and says to the steering wheel: 'You are stupid, why don't you turn round properly?' She mounts once more and rides down a slope. She tries without much success to use the brakes, tells the bicycle to stop and gets off again. Angrily, she strips a few grass blades from the lawn, just when the group of children flits by once more. At this point, 1-year-old Elisa appears holding her mother's hand tightly. Irina fetches the baby's large coloured ball and throws it towards her playfully, but is disappointed when the baby girl does not throw it back. Elisa picks up the ball and puts it to her ear. Her mother asks: 'What are you doing? Are you listening to the voice of the sea?' The baby girl is motionless, captivated and carried away by what she seems to hear with her ear stuck to the ball. Irina watches her intently and after a while asks Elisa with a timid smile whether she would let her hear too. She takes the ball, lifts it to her ear and stands listening for a while. Then, she gives it back to Elisa saying: 'I don't hear anything'. ('*Non sento niente*'. In Italian, there is only one verb – '*sentire*' – for both 'hearing' and 'feeling'.)

The 1-year-old Elisa seemed still to be able to enter a realm of sound-emotions or emotion-sounds and to have a blissful experience listening to the sounds in the ball, which the mother empathically knew about, as if in maternal reverie the curtain of amnesia could be temporarily lifted. But 4-year-old Irina had no access to this world any more and seemed to have become deaf to the sound of the sea.

Isaacs (1952: 105) writes:

When the visual elements in perception begin to predominate over the somatic . . . the concrete bodily elements . . . largely undergo *repression*. The visual . . . elements in phantasy become relatively de-emotionalized . . . independent, in consciousness, of bodily ties. They become 'images' in the narrower sense, representations 'in the mind' . . . It is realised that the objects are outside the mind, but their images are 'in the mind'. . . . Such images, however, draw their power . . . upon feelings, behaviour, character and personality, upon the mind as a whole, *from their repressed unconscious somatic associates* in the unconscious world of desire and emotions . . .

Auditory experience seems to be located at an intermediate level between the concrete world and imaginative thought. We have no difficulty in visualising an absent person or object by mental activity, but in order to evoke a melody clearly, most people have to sing it, which means the use of both mind and body.

Growth is not possible without repression, without loss and mourning. One of Piontelli's (1993: 14) observed children, a little girl of 4, helps her mother pick up the pieces of glass of a broken bottle. She knows that 'bottles break . . . and they cannot be put together again . . .'. Everyday life would be impracticable without the ability to forget and to relinquish memories of the past. But the roots of sound-emotions do not seem to disappear. Just as the 'unconscious somatic associates' (Isaacs 1952: 105) remain a source of power, sound-memories seem to animate and inspire our verbal language, if we allow them to do so. They emerge in song and music, in baby-talk, love-talk and poetry, but also, if we listen carefully enough, in everyday language.

THE SOUND-BREAST

A more detailed account of an infant observation describes a situation in which vocal interaction between the mother and the baby was particularly striking and important.

During the first telephone contact with the family, the observer was struck by the cheerfulness of the mother's voice. She also noted in her record that there was soft music in the background.

The interview took place a few days before delivery. The father was not present. The mother received the observer with great cordiality. The atmosphere in the house was calm and pleasant. Again, there was music in the background. The mother gave a detailed report of her pregnancy. She had suffered from nausea for the first four months and could not eat anything, but the following two months had been absolutely marvellous. She had never been so well in her life. While she said this, her face brightened up, and she offered the observer a drink. Her expression became tense again when she talked about the uterine contractions during the seventh month. She had spent three weeks in hospital, during which she was not allowed to move. But now, everything was fine again, and she felt ready for the baby to be born.

On the observer's first visit, Linda was three weeks old. The father was lying on the sofa, convalescent from a flu attack. He asked the observer many personal questions and then told her in detail the story of his wife's long and difficult delivery. The baby would not come out, and the obstetrician had considered the use of forceps. He himself appeared as the central figure in his account. The mother stood beside the sofa and smiled at him. Shortly before the end of the hour, she brought in Linda. The father thought she must be hungry, asked for the bottle and fed the baby, still lying on the sofa. The mother said sadly that she had no milk and could not breast-feed, but luckily her husband was very good at feeding the baby.

During the following weeks, the atmosphere was relaxed, and there was always soft background music. One day, Linda was lying in the cot and the mother was out of sight.

> At first, she remains quietly alert for some time, but then her limbs start stiffening, her back becomes rigid and her face red, and then, she expels a piercing cry. The mother talks to her softly from the distance, and Linda immediately relaxes at the sound of her voice. When the mother comes over to give her the dummy, the baby sucks it rhythmically for a while, but then opens her mouth, produces gurgling little sounds, and the dummy falls out. The mother responds with similar sounds and gives her the dummy back. Linda sucks only for a short moment, lets it go again and 'talks' as before, receiving a prompt echo from the mother's cheerful singsong.

There was strikingly less passion in Linda's relation with the bottle or the dummy than in the vocal interplay with her mother. She always sucked on the bottle quietly and without greed from the beginning of the feed. Every now and then, she paused, let the teat go and emitted gurgling sounds towards her mother. One day, Linda was in her mother's arms lalling and babbling. Her mother responded with the same tone of voice and said to the baby: 'Isn't this lovely music?' She then made a few dancing steps with her. They smiled lovingly at each other. This idyllic period coincided with the father's absence. He had gone abroad to visit his mother.

On the very day of his return, the mother, while feeding the baby, mentioned that she would resume work shortly. Linda did not seem to swallow properly, produced choking noises and contracted her face. The mother said that she would suffocate if she did not swallow, but did not withdraw the bottle. Linda panted and coughed until she managed to spit some milk.

Although the vocal interaction between the mother and the now two-and-a-half-months-old baby was as intense as ever, the observer was struck by the fact that Linda looked at her mother less, and often fixed on some point on the ceiling instead. The mother was puzzled too and tried to turn Linda's head towards her. The baby looked at her briefly and then fixed her gaze on the ceiling again and sometimes smiled and emitted sounds in that direction.

Linda was four months old when the mother went back to work. It was difficult to find a suitable time for the observation, and the father, who looked after the baby most of the time, made the observer feel unwanted and intrusive. He talked to Linda as if she were a much older child and tended to use her to show off his fathering capacities. He played eroticising games with her or offered her one object after the other in rapid sequence. She would try to put them in her mouth, but none of them ever fitted properly. They were either too hard or too square or too big.

The mother's attitude towards Linda changed. Their vocal interaction was still occasionally intense, but at times it was suddenly interrupted by orally aggressive episodes on the mother's part. She often adopted the father's mocking and denigrating attitudes, and there were occasions of actual gang-like collusion between the parents. In this period, the baby began having feeding difficulties. She refused to eat meat and fish and lived on milk and fruit.

When Linda was six months old, the observer began to worry because the baby made no attempts to crawl when put on her blanket on the floor. Sometimes, especially after she had been offered a hard or square toy that hurt when she tried to put it in her mouth, she stopped playing, her eyes fixed on to nowhere with a lost expression. On several occasions, the observer found the door locked and nobody at home.

Linda was eight months old when the observer saw her after one month's interruption for the holidays.

The baby looks at me again and again, with a serious expression. The mother comments that she cannot remember me, because she was a tiny baby when she last saw me. Linda is sitting on her mother's lap, and the father attracts her attention by calling her in a mockingly high-pitched witch-like tone. Although Linda is visibly frightened and buries her face in her mother's lap, the game is repeated several times.

This happened on the very day Linda had been with her childminder for the first time. She seemed to have cried for a long time, but at last she had fallen asleep with exhaustion. The father was satisfied with what he called the childminder's firmness. Linda's immobility was more and more striking. She sat still, her legs apart, her body sometimes oscillating to and fro and her eyes lost. She had one cold after the other, and the mother complained that she herself caught them from her daughter.

When Linda was nine months old, the mother was pregnant again. During the two following weeks, Linda's cough worsened dramatically, and two observations were cancelled. The observer was told later that Linda's breath had become rattling and her face had gone blue. Had they not taken her to the hospital, where bronchiolitis was diagnosed, she would have died of suffocation, the parents reported. When Linda was back home, she persisted in her immobile position or rocking movements, and now occasionally also made fluttering arm movements. Another crisis followed: a relapse of bronchiolitis and acute otitis media. This time, rapid medical intervention prevented a second hospitalisation. The father commented: 'a few more hours, and she would have been gone'. At this point, the mother's attitude changed. She said: 'It would have broken my heart to see her in hospital once more', and added, 'if I imagine not being able to breathe any more. . . . How terrible, isn't it, little one?' She hoped that this terrible experience would not have a negative influence on Linda's character. She took unpaid leave from work, so she could dedicate herself fully to the child. From that day, there were fewer verbal attacks from the father too. He was generally less present than before and often worked in his room, while the mother looked after the child. There were no more cancellations of observations.

At eleven months of age, Linda started crawling and exploring space. During a brief absence of her mother, the little girl looked for her teddy bear and did not give up until she found it. She lifted it up to her face and rocked it for a moment, then dropped it on the floor. When the mother came back, she welcomed her with a bright smile, said 'mammmma' and hid her smiling face in her mother's lap.

When Linda was 1 year, her babbling and vocalising became more and more modulated and articulate, while her relation both with the bottle and solid food tended to become less ambivalent. The child listened intently to her mother's communications and had an extraordinary capacity to reproduce the tone, rhythm and modulation of her voice.

One day, the mother comments that today Linda will go to sleep later than usual. She says, in a rhythmically swinging tone: '*Andrai a nanna più tardi.*' The child replies, with the same intonation: 'N*a*-ta, n*a*-ta'. And the mother confirms: 'Yes, that's right.'

At thirteen months of age, Linda pulled herself to her feet and made her first steps. When she looked at her books, she pointed at the animals and reproduced the voices with great competence. She clearly remembered the people, animals and places represented in the illustrations and was able to find them again. She also played hide-and-seek with the observer on her arrival. Separation now seemed to have become a bearable event. Linda was capable of thinking and naming the absent, especially her beloved grandfather and Laura, a little girl of her age, who used to come and play with her.

'A-u-l-a?', says Linda, echoing her mother's words. The mother replies: 'Yes, Laura went home to have a nap'. With the same questioning tone, Linda repeats: 'A-u-l-a?' and points her finger at the corridor. The mother says: 'Yes, Laura has gone home.' Linda crawls to the main door, and mother confirms that Laura will come back tomorrow.

The mother's pregnancy proceeded, and Linda asked her over and over again to read books about births and babies.

She looks at a book with her mother. There is a big apple and a little worm that crawls out of it. 'A little worm just like you', says the mother. Linda indicates the hole out of which it comes, and then the whole apple. Then, she slides down from her mother's lap and crawls away, as if she really were the little worm herself. When I am about to leave, Linda swiftly hides under the table and from this protected place waves good-bye to me.

The mother herself seemed to have a great need to talk with the observer about the approaching birth. When Linda found the image of the baby in the book, she pointed at her mother's body. The dialogue between mother and child was as intense as it had been at the beginning of Linda's life. The mother promptly verbalised her gestures, facial expressions and vocal messages, and Linda repeated the mother's words in an ongoing, reciprocally confirming, meaning-giving dialogue.

Mother and child look at a photo album. Linda has learned very quickly to recognise people, particularly the pictures of herself as a baby. She pronounces her name and expects the mother to repeat and confirm her identity. When the album is almost finished, Linda says: '*Giù*' (down), slides from her mother's lap, climbs on the sofa and sits next to her, leaning her head tenderly against her arm. It is as if she both re-experienced her own separation from her mother and anticipated her baby brother's birth.

Shortly before the mother's delivery, Linda had breathing difficulties again, but this time they were containable and seemed to be not much more than a tearless sobbing, when she clung to her mother's legs and would not let her go.

> Two days before her little brother is born, Linda touches her mother's pregnant body and says: '*Bibo*' (*bimbo*, child). She then goes over to the cot, which has been prepared for the new baby and looks into it. She goes to and fro many times between the cot and her mother, who confirms again and again that the little brother will sleep in the cot when he has come out, and that Linda has been in there too when she was a tiny baby. Linda repeats her own name and the word for cot. Then, she goes out on the balcony, from where the voices of playing children can be heard. She crouches, holds on to the bars of the railing and says '*bibi*' (*bimbi*, children) while watching the children play out there in the open.

DISCUSSION

Many painful events occurred in Linda's first year of life, and it was amazing to see her capacity not only to survive mentally, but also to go through actual life-threatening experiences, recovering an apparently undamaged capacity for hope and growth. She was not safely contained in her mother's womb during pregnancy. There had been a danger of premature birth. Her mother's breasts never gave her nourishment, and Linda missed the experience of a gratifying fit between mouth and nipple. Furthermore, her father's mind not only did not hold her, but exposed her actively to the sufferings of his own unhappy childhood. But the adults' collusion in projecting into the baby both the anxieties they were unable to tolerate themselves and their unintegrated aggressive feelings, was more than she could bear. After the mother's return to work, which coincided with her spending the day with the severe childminder, and also with the onset of the mother's second pregnancy, Linda fell ill. Her stay in hospital brought about yet another experience of abandonment. In the mother's mind, the hospital was connected both with the threat of Linda's premature expulsion during her pregnancy, and with the long and difficult labour when she withheld the baby and could not let her go. It is not surprising that Linda would not move on her carpet when she was back home.

But what seems particularly striking is the fact that Linda's illness had to do with breathing and sounds. Her lively babbling and vocalising was dramatically transformed into a choking cough and rattling breath, and she could have died of suffocation. When Bion (1963: 95) describes the mind's thought-transforming function, he uses the metaphor of the digestive tube. And he goes on suggesting that the respiratory and the auditory system could analogously be seen as models for the transformation of feelings. Linda had manifested her distress in both her respiratory and auditory organs when she fell ill with bronchiolitis and otitis media.

Precisely these two organs had been involved when she was a little baby; when she smiled, babbled and vocalised, and showed in many ways that her most intense experiences of interaction with her mother were auditory and vocal. Her feeding experience had not been such as to allow her to introject a harmonious reciprocity between the mouth and the nipple. Sounds seemed to fit her ears and mouth better than the hard toys she was offered, and better also than the dummy or the teat. We can wonder how the immateriality of sounds can fulfil in part the function of the concrete firmness and resilience of the nipple, but it is a fact that after the worrying signs of emotional retreat and her illnesses, which brought about her mother's and to some extent her father's emotional growth, Linda recovered surprisingly well, and her development moved on again. Her inner objects after all seemed to be reliable enough for her to be able, in a very short time span, to accept getting down from her mother's lap, to stand on her own feet and even to think about the birth of her baby brother.

Linda's mental activity, her memory and rapidity of language development were amazing. It is probable that it was rooted in the ground of the intense vocal interplay between her mother and herself in the very first months of her life. As to the pre-natal roots of her good object, we cannot go any further than state that the time of marvellous well-being described by her mother during the fifth and sixth month of pregnancy coincides with the period when the foetus's hearing capacity is fully developed. The introjection of the mother's voice during the emotionally intense vocal interaction at the beginning of Linda's extra-uterine life may have contributed in helping her to get over the crisis of her illness. If there is something like a sound-object with pre-natal roots, we may wonder whether it could even have had some sustaining and life-maintaining function at the time of the threat of the child's premature birth.

CONCLUSION

The examples of vocal interaction between mother and infant were used to show how much of the emotional quality of their relation is expressed at a sound-level, and therefore how important the sound-aspect of inner objects can be. Possibly, this interplay is influenced by both the baby's and the mother's pre-natal auditory experiences. We have seen in Linda's observation material how competent infants can be in clinging to one mode of interaction, especially if the others are for some reason insufficient, and still be able to create in themselves a wholeness of experience. Before birth, when the visual elements are practically non-existent, the auditory experience is the only way of sensing distance and otherness. While taste and tactile experiences are synonymous with presence, the unborn infant's hearing capacity is somehow the extreme outpost of the possibility of experiencing absence and thus otherness, and can therefore be thought to be located at the very root of symbolisation. Mother's voice, in fact, is beyond the child's power to reproduce and may hence, when she is silent, bring about the first experience of an unreachable desired object, in other words, the precursor of the post-natal 'no-breast' experience.

In relation to infant observation, it seems important to pay particular attention not only to visual and verbal aspects, but also to sound-elements; not only because it allows us, from a general point of view, to have a more global perception of things, but because the sound-contents in the material confront observers more consciously with the deepest aspects of their own early experiences. This does not mean an attempt to overcome the barrier of infantile amnesia, but to heighten the sensitivity towards the manifestations of possible pre-natal memories, and deepen the insight into their meaning, which is often concealed in rhythms, sounds and voices. Special attention to sounds can enhance the 'light of the ears'.

REFERENCES

Bion, W. R. (1963) *Elements of Psychoanalysis*, London: Heinemann.
Brazelton, T. B. (1973) *Neonatal Behavioral Assessment Scale*, London: Heinemann, and Philadelphia: Lippincott Co.
Isaacs, S. (1952) 'The nature and function of phantasy', in J. Riviere (ed.) *Developments in Psychoanalysis*, London: Hogarth.
Maiello, S. (1995) 'The sound-object', *Journal of Child Psychotherapy*, 21, 1: 23–41 (first published as 'L'oggetto sonoro', *Richard e Piggle*, 1, 1: 31–47, Roma: Il Pensiero Scientifico, 1993).
Meltzer, D. *et al.* (1986) *Studies in Extended Metapsychology*, Strath Tay, Perthshire: Clunie Press.
Piontelli, A. (1992) *From Fetus to Child, An Observational and Psychoanalytical Study*, London: Routledge.
Piontelli, A. (1993) 'Some reflections on infantile amnesia', *The British Psychoanalytical Bulletin*, 29,1: 11–18.
Prechtl, H. F. R. (1989) 'Fetal behaviour', in A. Hill and J. Volpe (eds) *Fetal Neurology*, New York: Raven Press.
Schneider, M. (1992) *La musica primitiva*, Milano: Adelphi (first published as *Le rôle de la musique dans la mythologie et les rites des civilisations non européennes*, Paris: Gallimard, 1960).
Tomatis, A. (1987) *Der Klang des Lebens*, Reinbek bei Hamburg: Rowohlt Verlag (first published as *La nuit utérine*, Paris: Editions Stock, 1981).

Part III

Research developments

Introduction

Susan Reid

Infant observation has been undertaken primarily for training purposes, rather than research. However, from the outset the observations have been conducted in accordance with a standardised protocol and recorded in considerable detail.

Nowadays, up to 125 such observations are undertaken in any one year under the auspices of Tavistock Clinic training programmes alone. The numbers of infants being observed in many trainings, in different cultural settings, around the world, is incalculable. All these observations constitute a significant database of research material, which has not yet been utilised on a significant scale for research purposes. Experienced child development researchers have also recognised that this constitutes a considerable unutilised research resource, especially since the method of writing up these observations has required observational and narrative description, largely uncontaminated, at the data collection and recording stage, by theoretical conceptualisation.

In parallel, in the last twenty years there has been a rapid growth of more experimental and laboratory-based research into infant development, some of which has been quite convergent with the approaches of psychoanalysis (e.g. Stern 1985; Trevarthen 1977, 1979, 1980; Murray 1991). Within the related tradition of Attachment Theory, deriving from the work of John Bowlby (1969) and Mary Ainsworth *et al.* (Ainsworth 1969; Ainsworth *et al.* 1978), methodologies have been developed, especially the 'Strange Situation Test', which have enabled standardised observations to be made of large numbers of infants.

A conference in 1994, initiated by Professor Michael Rustin, a sociologist with a particular interest in psychoanalysis, brought together the attachment theorists, Mary Main and Eric Hesse, with Tavistock-trained infant observers. The comparison of the two methodologies proved stimulating. The attachment theory tradition has developed powerful empirical tools, invaluable in clinical research, but it is acknowledged that in so doing the complex and differentiated descriptions of infant development and family interactions yielded by the psychoanalytic method, has, of necessity, been sacrificed.

The psychoanalytic approach has not yet developed more systematic classifying, coding and verification procedures which would enable the information provided by the individual case studies to be analysed in a more systematic and comparative way. The findings from infant observation studies have long informed a wide range of clinical research projects and influenced clinical practice, contributions to psychoanalytic thinking and decisions to explore particular areas in clinical research. However, we have largely failed to find a way to share the research potential with colleagues of other disciplines and traditions of thinking. It is hoped that this section of the book will help to redress this omission.

We have now begun to explore the more formal research potential of this methodology. More recent works, making use of individual observational case studies, have sought to demonstrate, using empirical observational evidence, how this contribution can be developed. Piontelli, for example, in her work (Piontelli 1992) has explored the use of infant observation to inform our understanding of the experience of the foetus, and how foetal experiences influence subsequent developments in the infant after birth.

Michael Rustin in the book *Closely Observed Infants* (Miller *et al.* 1989) discusses infant observation as a method of research. Rustin contends that there is 'scope for adapting this observational method for a more focused study of infancy'. Current clinical trainings are increasingly seeking a link to academic institutions. This has encouraged the development of research as a component of the training. The next generation of clinicians are therefore increasingly likely to be trained researchers.

This section of the book outlines two infant observation research studies. Both studies, using small samples, explore the value of the qualitative research method. The importance of laboratory-based research projects has already been recognised together with their limitations. The limitations of qualitative research are well known. These two studies reveal something of the richness of information the methodology yields, along with a recognition of the difficulties inherent in operationalising some of the more abstract concepts of psychoanalytic theory necessary to facilitate comparisons between infants.

In Chapter 11, 'Observed families revisited – two years on: a follow-up study', Gertraud Diem-Wille outlines her methodology devised to test out the validity and reliability of the observational data gathered in the ordinary course of events in any infant observation. In her study she followed up four infants, two girls and two boys, two years after the conclusion of the initial observations, drawing on the data collected by the original observer and from interviews with each observer. If the method is valid, then the patterns of development described by the

observer should allow for hypotheses to be made about future development. Diem-Wille uses one of her subjects, Kelly, to describe her
methodology in detail, demonstrating the convergence between the hypotheses she made, based on her original observational data, with her own
subsequent observations of the child at 4 years of age.

The role and impact of the observer on the infant and family observed
is frequently a focus for discussion. It has become apparent that for most
families the impact of the observer has been benign and even sometimes
therapeutic. Some families have even requested a second observer for
their next baby. Diem-Wille also sets out to test the impact of the observer
in a more rigorous way. Central to the hypothesis is the idea that in the
process of an observation the observer is actually containing some of
the elements in the relationships within a family which cannot be thought
about by the families themselves (see Chapter 7).

In the interviews with the parents, the very openness with which they
speak and their willingness to take part, seem to pay tribute to the largely
benign experience of being observed. It is clear that they expect to be
thought about respectfully by the new observer and there is an obvious
expectation that they will not be judged. This allows for considerable
honesty when reflecting upon a period in the family's life which was
distressing as well as pleasurable.

This small study substantiates the experiences informally gathered by
individual infant observers, seminar groups and those who have taught
this method of study for many years. Within any infant observation group
hypotheses are constantly made and tested. Patterns in development
emerge, some stronger than others. Some patterns appear more susceptible
to change and influence than others. Diem-Wille's study supports the
central notion that good observational detail can provide the information
necessary for making hypotheses.

The link between Diem-Wille's study and the work of Piontelli is
interesting. Piontelli's work has taken us backwards in time to experiences
before birth. Her twin studies suggest that experiences *in utero* are predictive of development after birth. Diem-Wille's study supports the notion
that experiences in early infancy can be predictive of subsequent development. This study paves the way for large-scale longitudinal studies
following some observed infants into adulthood.

In Chapter 12, 'Observing when infants are at potential risk: reflections
from a study of five infants, concentrating on observations of a Bengali
infant', Dr Briggs focuses on the role of observation as a research tool.
Setting out to observe five infants on a weekly basis, each of whom was
designated 'at risk', he explores the relationship between the observer, the
observed infants and their families. Because he was obliged to adopt a
more interventionist approach than is usually the case, due to the 'at risk'

situations of the infants observed, his chapter illuminates the containing function of the observer.

In Briggs's study he explores the nature of the containment available to the infants and its impact upon their subsequent development. In this chapter he focuses upon one of the infants, Hashmat, and the defences he employs against the lack of containment available to him. The cultural differences between the observed and the observer make a strong link to Chapter 4. In the lack of integration between eye contact and mouth grip observed in Hashmat, there is a fascinating link to Chapter 9.

The study gives an insight into life in a large family, common enough after all in most cultures before the advent of birth control. Reading this study is a useful reminder that the small nuclear family only goes back a generation or two. Our own historical backgrounds will soon reveal a family of similar size to Hashmat's. The observational material allows us to empathise more closely with situations which may be at variance with current experiences of family life for many readers, but which may have had some influence upon us through intergenerational patterns of child-rearing.

The vivid quality of the observational material allows the reader a first-hand understanding of the need for the 'group' to take on some of the parenting tasks in such a large family. It becomes easy to sympathise with the challenging task for any mother and father trying to create mental space, to be receptive and emotionally available to so many disparate needs. Turning to the family group can therefore be seen as an appropriate variation in style of parenting from that which is known most intimately in modern Western societies.

It is clear that within such a large family group other children will often resent the requirement for them to parent their younger siblings. The excerpts from the observations allow the reader some insight into why certain characterological traits may predominate in some large families. We see Hashmat, who has been the victim of his older siblings' aggression, in turn take on the role of the aggressor in relation to the new baby in the family. Here the new baby is a real threat to the older siblings who experience insufficient nurturing of their emotional needs. An aggressive response in these circumstances may be more readily understood.

Some emotional toughness seems to be required to survive life in a large family where the emotional resources of any parents would be over-stretched. Perhaps individuality can only be nurtured and valued in those societies which no longer require large families to ensure the survival of the species. Survival can here be understood to mean the survival of cultural identity in a host culture where racism is a fact of daily life.

In our current infant observation studies, where most of the families consist of only two or three children, we are impressed by those parents who cope imaginatively and thoughtfully with the often conflicting needs of children born close together. The impossibility of sustaining a thoughtful contact in a large family becomes extremely apparent. The drive to 'switch off' can be seen as not pathological but an essential defence. We gain a real insight into what it can be like to grow up in such a large family *regardless* of race or culture. It confronts us with the realities of such a situation and prevents us from any unhelpful wish to romanticise the delights of being one of a large family. The particularly shocking incident when Hashmat is exposed to the violence of a resentful sibling thus takes on a universality.

Ultimately one is left deeply impressed by Hashmat's resilience – his capacity to be loving and thoughtful is shown to have survived, although his identification with the aggressor gives cause for concern. The testament to the containing role of the observer is eloquently made by Hashmat himself in the final observation when he raises his glass to Dr Briggs and says 'Cheers!'

Briggs's research produced a wealth of material which is not only rich in its own right but also stimulates ideas for other research studies. Hashmat's failure to grow in his early months gives an interesting perspective on some 'failure to thrive infants' and opens up another area for further exploration. As indicated by this study, there is enormous potential for the comparison of other groups of infants such as blind and adopted babies.

REFERENCES

Ainsworth, Mary D. Salter (1969) 'Object relations, dependency and attachment: a theoretical review of the infant-mother relationship', *Child Development*, 40: 969–1025.
Ainsworth, M., Blehar, M. C., Waters, E. and Wall, S. (1978) *Patterns of Attachment: A Psychological Study of the Strange Situation*, Hillsdale, NJ.: Lawrence Erlbaum.
Bowlby, J. (1969) *Attachment and Loss*, Vol. 1, London Hogwarth Press.
Miller, L., Rustin, M. and Shuttleworth, J. (1989) *Closely Observed Infants*, London: Duckworth.
Murray, L. (1991) 'Intersubjectivity, object relations theory and empirical evidence from mother-infant interactions', *Infant Mental Health Journal*, 12: 219–232.
Piontelli, A. (1992) *From Fetus to Child: An Observational and Psychoanalytic Study*, London: Tavistock/Routledge.
Stern, D. (1985) *The Interpersonal World of the Infant*, New York: Basic Books
Trevarthen, Colwyn (1977) 'Descriptive analyses of infant communicative behaviour', in H. R. Schaffer (ed.) *Studies in Mother–Infant Interaction*, pp. 227–70, London: Academic Press.
Trevarthen, Colwyn (1979) 'Infant play and the creation of culture', *New Scientist*, 81: 566–569.
Trevarthern, Colwyn (1980) 'Foundations of intersubjectivity: development of interpersonal and co-operative understanding of infants', in D. Olson (ed.) *The Social Foundations of Language and Thought*, New York: W. W. Norton.

Chapter 11

Observed families revisited – two years on

A follow-up study

Gertraud Diem-Wille

This chapter describes a research project I undertook during a sabbatical year spent at the Tavistock Clinic. I arrived as an interested but sceptical psychologist, having first encountered infant observation in Vienna, where a small group had recently formed to explore the potential of the method. My project was planned to investigate two main questions, although other themes also emerged. I was interested in devising a methodology which would test out the validity and reliability of observational data gathered within the naturalistic frame of ordinary infant observation practice, and of the psychoanalytically based interpretation of this data, which provides an account of a child's personal development and explores qualities of transgenerational patterns. I also wished to find out what parents felt about the experience of having an observer in the family. I shall first describe the methodology I adopted, then present a detailed case study, and finally draw together some conclusions.

During my stay at the Tavistock Clinic as a 'Visiting Scientist' attached to the Child and Family Department, I started to learn about infant observation and the counselling service for the parents of babies and young children. I was deeply impressed by the elaborate method of infant observation introduced in 1948 by Esther Bick and by the enormous amount of data already collected with research potential.

I encountered colleagues keen to support a research project and interested in the questions I was raising: How might it be possible to check the validity of the descriptive material and of the psychoanalytical interpretation of the material in the seminars which accompany the observations? Does infant observation enable one to measure and understand the patterns of communication and the unconscious aspects of the relationships in the family? Do the student observers collect data which provide significant insight into the inner world of the baby and thus explore the core of the developing personality of the child?

My intention was to go back to children who had been observed as infants and compare the description of the child built up during the two-year observation with a follow-up observation two or three years later. I thus defined infant observation not only as a training method but also as a research method to collect data about a family.

The sample for the follow-up study was chosen from infant observations undertaken by students at the Tavistock Clinic. It consisted of firstborn children (two of each gender) and their parents, where the student who had done the observation was still available for consultation. The design consisted of four steps:

1 Reading the paper written at the end of the observation and formulating hypotheses about future lines of personality development;
2 Doing an interview with the student observer about their perception of the observation, and asking for comments about the predictions about the child made by the researcher;
3 Being introduced to the originally observed family by the student. I asked whether they would consent to take part in the study, which would mean being observed a few times at home plus an additional observation in a different setting, such as playgroup or school, to get a second impression of the child's social behaviour outside the family. If the parents were separated, I suggested an observation of the child with the parent no longer living at home.
4 Doing an interview with each parent separately, where they were asked about their views of the observation, how they experienced the pregnancy and birth, and about their relationship with their own parents when they were children.

The research material was discussed with an experienced infant observation teacher, Margaret Rustin, and her helpful comments and thoughts are integrated in my account.

A qualitative approach seemed to me the most appropriate model for understanding the development of a child. My design, based on seeing the family at home, fits with a central idea in qualitative research which emphasises the values of the natural environment, in contrast to the controlled experimental situation in a laboratory, since the former can provide richer results and more realistic information. Experiments in laboratories:

> are tighter and more rigorous and give rise to more reliable data, replicable effects and a claim to greater objectivity. However, results are open to the criticism of giving narrow, unrealistic information using measures which trap only a tiny portion of the concept originally under study.

> (Coolican 1970: 38).

An experimental design reduces the richness of a parent-infant relationship to a specific interaction. For example, when Mary Ainsworth developed the experiment to assess the attachment of a child to its parents, the measure was the infant's stranger and separation anxiety in a laboratory where the observation is controlled through the structure of the experiment. Using infant observation as a method of collecting data by observing a relatively unconstrained segment of a person's freely chosen behaviour and the interaction in the family, means also that the research produces unpredictable amounts and types of information which the researcher has to sift, organise and select for significance. This method leaves the researcher more room to manoeuvre in questioning the participants and in deciding what observations yield interpretations of interest. The price is a greater individual or family-system bias and less comparability between studies.

I will now proceed to a case study of one of the families with whom I negotiated the research intervention described above.

A CASE STUDY: KELLY

The structure of the case presentation follows the research design, starting with the implicit hypotheses about the observed infant and then comparing them with the data I obtained from my own observation of the family and from the interview with the parents.

In the infant observation paper, which is based on a weekly one-hour observation over two years, the student tries to summarise the recurrent patterns in the relationship of mother and baby to allow the individual character of the baby to emerge. There is no given structure which would enable one to compare different papers. Each is unique and different in its attempt to synthesise the complex situation in a family. I tried to identify seven *dimensions* which are relevant for the development of the child's personality. The first four dimensions concern the child's inner reality:

1 The balance between good internal objects and idealized or persecutory objects;
2 Stimulating and deprived aspects of the environment;
3 The balance between primitive and more mature defences;
4 Containing, as contrasted with intrusive and inconsistent aspects of mother.

The last three dimensions arise from the parental interviews and the observed attitude of parents to their child:

5 Setting and negotiating rules versus inflexible rules or none;
6 Acknowledgement and encouragement versus inhibition of the child's development;
7 Good social skills and sensitivity versus little social contact.

In making predictions about Kelly's future development, we need to remain aware of the fact that, although the early experiences in life form a core of a personality, the events of outer reality (for example parental divorce, socio-economic situation, a new partnership, birth of a sibling, etc.) have a major impact on a child. Furthermore, adolescence is crucial for the final structuring of psychic reality. Freud wrote:

> The first of these developments begins between the age of two and five, and is brought to a halt or to a retreat by the latency period. . . . The second wave sets in with puberty and determines the final outcome of sexual life.
>
> (Freud 1905: 200)

As Margot Waddell puts it, 'adolescence offers a second opportunity to engage with experiences and possible developments which were not available earlier, whether for reasons of health, loss, separation, or other problems' (Waddell 1994: 55). It would therefore be interesting to review Kelly's development at a later point.

Kelly in the two-year observation: extracts from the observational record

Let me start with the description of the family as it is given in the original paper. The parents are described as an older, middle-class married couple, very polite, warm and humorous. The parents had moved into their house at the beginning of the pregnancy, in a fairly quiet street in a busy city suburb. Both were looking forward to having a baby. They also seem to have a secure financial situation. Mother went back to part-time work when Kelly was four months old and to full-time work when Kelly was nine months old. She appeared efficient, well-organised and controlled.

Kelly was born three weeks premature and her weight at birth was seven pounds and four ounces. Mother was well-prepared for a natural birth by attending yoga and National Child Birth Trust classes, but as the labour was long and painful she decided to take Pethedine.

Hypothesis 1

The overall impression transmitted in the paper is that Mother is able to provide a secure and stable relationship, holding the baby close, and breast-feeding her, and is able to receive the infant's signals and understand them. From the first observation Kelly reacts to Mother's voice, she 'relaxed visibly when Mother answered the phone'. One could interpret that Kelly is psychically 'held together' by her mother's voice which represents mother's aliveness. Kelly is described as an active, responsive baby. So when we take into consideration Kelly's innate endowment or temperament she could be called an 'easy baby', a category into which 50 per cent of all babies fall, according to Thomas and Chess (1977), when they are 'moderately active and innately adaptable'.

Mother can wait until Kelly is definitely hungry and expresses her hunger with a distinctive cry, and does not use the breast as a response to every kind of distress. This leads me to an hypothesis on my first dimension.

Kelly has developed a good internal object that enables her to establish a secure relationship and forms a stable base to cope with problems and to develop a solid self-esteem.

There is one scene when Kelly is separated from her parents when both of them leave the room, she complains and shows her unhappiness.

When both her parents left the room she looked after them in a concerned manner and uttered short urgent cries until Mother asked Father to return. When Father sat down Kelly became quiet, and looked from Father to me as she sat on the floor.

This description reminds me of the 'Strange Situation' experiment by Mary Ainsworth (Ainsworth *et al.* 1978), studying the reaction of 1-year-old to separation in a laboratory situation. Kelly shows the reaction that is ascribed to secure attached children. Such children show their anger, anxiety and distress and cry because they have the experience that their parents will not leave them. They trust their parents to come back if they cry.

Hypothesis 2

From the very beginning there is respect for the personality of the baby. She has space to explore toys and later, when she can move around, she crawls around in the room with her mother staying in the room and watching over her. Kelly seems to be perceived as an autonomous unique being and is encouraged to have her own experiences as a separate person. She has a lot of books and all three grown-ups in her life like to read them to her, so she gets a lot of stimulation and prompting. The observer writes:

Kelly is a bright, lively little girl with ready curiosity about her. She has brown hair and brown eyes. She is slim and agile. She explores all the corners of the room in her play. Her smile is broad and infectious. She has a gutsy laugh and a great sense of humour. She enjoys involving adults in her play and reading her books with someone while sucking her thumb in concentration. She also can be quite absorbed by herself sitting quietly and thoughtfully, or intensely working on something as she plays.

Mother and probably Father provided a safe and stimulating environment that helped her to develop her ability to symbolise and play in a creative way. Language and music seemed to be her favourite way of expressing herself and of making contact with her parents. One can expect her to be curious and exploratory, open to learning and conceptualising.

Hypothesis 3

Another important structure of the personality is the way in which unbearable impulses are dealt with. What defence mechanisms do we see during the observation?

The observer described how Kelly coped with the separation from Mother when she went back to work. 'Kelly appeared quite uncontrollable in her distress and her frantic search for Mother's breast.' The observer is inclined to understand the long continuation of breast-feeding (two years) as a way of compensating for mother's absence for five days a week when she works, and as a sign of the guilt she feels in leaving the baby with the nanny. But we could also surmise that Baby and Mother need the protective closeness of the breast-feeding in the morning and in the evening.

Often Kelly is very excited and agitated 'like an actress'.

Kelly became known from an early age for being an actress. Mother remarked on her strong and independent will and her attempt to show off and play for rewarding laughs and smiles by the way she made funny noises and faces.

The observer interprets it later: 'There is an idea in the description of actress of somehow not being real, and some distance between fantasy and reality.' Can we understand this description of Kelly as a generosity of spirit and openness, or is there also a hint of a show element in her? Is she supplying something for the grown-ups to entertain them and cheer them up?

Kelly has a tendency to cover deep feelings, loss and separation behind manic hyperactivity and exciting games. This might enable her to use her abilities and talents partly in a constructive and partly in a defensive way.

Hypothesis 4

It was suggested that the long breast-feeding could be partly connected with Kelly's wish to control the breast but also with mother's wish to be unique, in other words, as mother's idealisation of the breast. When Kelly was eighteen months old, Mother had told the observer that she had tried to wean her and she wrote:

Kelly was most insistent that the breast should be available to her on Mother's return from work, as if this might allow her phantasies of controlling the breast to be fulfilled. Yet there remains the question of Mother's ambivalence, not wishing to prevent Kelly from enjoying this reunion . . . but also perhaps the feeling she still has a special place that no-one else could fill.

Could it therefore also be that subconsciously Kelly knows she has to look after Mother and wants to keep her happy by needing her so close for such a long time? This would mean that Kelly develops a capacity to cheer Mother up and give emotional meaning to Mother's life. We would then expect Kelly to behave in a nice, grown-up way in order to please Mother.

We also see that Mother feels easily rejected by Kelly when she bites her bib or her teething ring. We read, 'Mother commented on Kelly perhaps preferring these things to the food she gives her and preferring Daddy to Mummy.'

Kelly introjects Mother's wish to be unique and special and looks after Mother to protect her vulnerability. We expect her to be partly a parent-ified child, i.e., she suppresses her own feelings and needs in order to protect her mother.

Hypothesis 5

If we look for examples of how the parents negotiate problems and find solutions, we find a quite flexible approach. Mother and maybe also Father do not get stuck in battles with Kelly but work out solutions. When Mother postponed feeding solids because Kelly had objected, it might be partly because she wanted to keep the breast as something special, but she also conveyed the message that the child's reaction is taken into consideration.

Kelly will be a child who expects explanations and will fight to get her way, but will provide a range of possible solutions or compromises when she negotiates with somebody. She will be flexible and imaginative in finding ways of being heard and considered. In combination with her omnipotent, controlling side she might do it in a manipulative way, using her charm and humour to get what she wants. (This contrasts with the previous hypothesis.)

Hypothesis 6

Kelly not only gets a lot of stimulation from her parents but also from her grandmother and other children.

Kelly was interested in Mother's body, she played with Mother's body and buried her face in Mother's breast. She also played with a little figure in the box.

This would show that Kelly was able to symbolise 'her worries about another baby in Mother's body in a playful way'. The observer refers to the relationship between Grandmother and Kelly as 'warm and easy':

> I remember particularly how she would arrive from work and pick Kelly up and read through a book with such imagination in her voice and in her manner that thoroughly enthralled Kelly. It seemed to make a contrast to the more uncertain attitude that Mother had. Sometimes she took it personally when Kelly lost interest.

Grandmother seems to be lively and outgoing with a lot of imagination that she can share with Kelly.

Kelly will have a wide range of interests and goals and will pursue them with pleasure and joy. It could also help her to gain gratification. As she gains acknowledgement for her broad interests, this will create a benign circle. This mutual reinforcement will become more varied and complex with increased skills and strategies.

Hypothesis 7

Kelly had to cope from an early age with different childminders, so she learned to discriminate between different situations and people. We learn how stimulated Kelly was by the presence of another child. When he came, she was not yet able to walk.

> As soon as Paul joined her, Kelly was on her feet. Kelly on the whole enjoyed the presence of the other children and played many cooperative games. However, it also became quickly apparent that there was a great deal of rivalry. It was usually Kelly, at least in the early weeks of the nanny-sharing arrangements, who had the toy or object that was suddenly greatly desired by him. Paul would try and pull it from her. At first Kelly seemed indifferent to letting things go. She did after all have her familiar containing house and toys around her . . . Kelly showed her authority and at times literally walked over him.

One must keep in mind that both children were playing in Kelly's house, so we can suppose that she considered him as an intruder in her home, and she had to share Nanny with him.

Kelly will make use of social situations and enjoy the company of others. She is likely to try to be the centre of attention but to remain sensitive to the social context.

These seven dimensions of Kelly's personality cannot be considered as strictly separate. On the contrary, they influence each other.

Kelly two years later

I then used these dimensions to study the data of the follow-up observation undertaken when Kelly was 4 years old. I was able to observe Kelly twice with her mother and once with her father. The situation of Kelly's parents had changed totally. The parents separated when Kelly was eighteen months old. She now lives with her mother but has regular contact with her father. She visits him every other weekend and stays overnight once a month. Kelly started school when she was 4 years old. I shall now use my seven hypotheses as a basis for my comments.

Hypothesis 1: Good versus idealized or persecutory internal objects

There was a lot of physical contact between Mother and Kelly. When Mother talked to me, Kelly leaned against her and Mother stroked her head. Kelly was attentive and picked up every idea Mother gave her. This is a sequence from the second observation.

> In her room Kelly went straight to her plastic play house which was full of different dolls and other toys. She took out a doll, told me her name and put it in the cot. When she passed by, she looked at me and said, 'Let's play mother, father, child. I'm the mother and you are father.' Without expecting an answer, she talked to the little doll like a mother to her child, holding it close to her head, laughing and talking to her about how her day had been and how things were. She lay down the doll carefully, covered it with a blanket and went back to take out a teddy bear.

When she is the mother of her doll she shows that she is identified with her caring mother. As her mother will go away the next morning, she also seems to be the doll and is in touch with her baby feelings. She may also thus symbolise that she is looking after herself. As Anne Alvarez points out: 'The imagination is the great healing ground and the great area of potential development' (Alvarez 1992: 81). In the observation with Father, Kelly showed that she had a strong and reliable relationship with him. This is an extract from the very beginning:

> Father told me they were in the middle of a story. He sat down on the sofa, Kelly cuddled close to Father purring gently. He put his arms around her, she had her face on his chest and he started to read. It seemed to be a familiar situation for both of them. Father has a deep and pleasant voice, he read the story like a radio play, imitating different persons, whispering sometimes in Kelly's ear. . . . She snuggled her face close to Daddy's chest while he was reading and turned her head towards me and gave me a big smile and I smiled back.

When Father is reading to her it is clearly a three-person situation – they both invited me to share the pleasure of reading. It is as if Kelly takes me as a substitute for a mother who lets them be together and can keep some distance. It is a relaxed and happy atmosphere and I do not feel excluded.

As we never have a direct access to the internal world and the way Kelly experiences her internal objects, we can only interpret her behaviour. When she plays at being a mother for her doll it suggests that she has in her internal world a concept of a mother who is looking after a child. She was able to cope with the upsetting divorce of her parents and she can provide inner space for both households.

Hypothesis 2: Stimulating versus deprived environment

In all three observations there are many examples of how she can use her imagination in play, invent new rules, be creative. She is aware of her wishes and has lots of ideas. There is also a lovely capacity to deal with new things. She giggles and enjoys games. I want to show in detail how she uses her imaginative and creative ability to cope with anxiety. During the observation with Father she showed me her room with a poster on the door saying: KELLY'S ROOM. MONSTERS KEEP OUT. When I asked her what it meant she explained it and went to the kitchen to draw me a picture:

> While she was drawing Father asked her what it was. It was a figure with some extensions. She explained which part was the head, then described each bit as she drew; the eyes, the nose, and the mouth. He asked whether it was a nice monster, she said 'No, a bad one', but laughed cheerfully. Then she drew a spider which looked more like a flower and said the monster would eat it. Father explained to her that a spider had eight legs and was black, he took a black pen and drew it in one corner. Kelly watched him, laughed, waited until he had finished, helping him count as he drew the legs and then, crossing it out with a red crayon, she explained that the monster would eat it. Father also enjoyed the game and asked her whether he should draw another spider. She nodded and he did another one in the other corner. And again it was eaten by the monster. So Father, encouraged by Kelly's response, suggested he would draw a big one, a huge one. He took a purple crayon and made a big one. She watched him with interest, waited until he had finished and said, 'Look what I'm doing now!' While she said this, she took the pen he had used before and drew over it and said this one was also eaten by the monster. But Father protested and said it was too big, the mouth of the monster wasn't big enough. But Kelly just laughed and made the mouth bigger. When Father said, 'It's not big enough' she made a huge mouth.

This sequence shows how Kelly is allowed to share her fantasy world with her father and they both enjoy it. In a way they do the drawing together. This spider-monster might be understood as her angry feelings. However, the monster can devour the spiders and so get rid of persecutors. Or if we interpret it in the context of Oedipal issues, it can be understood as a symbol referring to sexual intercourse with dominating oral phantasies. Kelly had told me that monsters are so hungry they could eat any spider. The big mouth of the monster in the later stage also expresses Kelly's anxiety about being eaten by the monster. She gave me this drawing as a present, thus she included me and my presence makes it probably more acceptable for her to be with her father.

Hypotheses 3 and 4: Primitive versus more mature defences, and Containing versus intrusive or inconsistent mothering

One moment when I experienced a strong projection into me is also connected with her wish to include Father in her play with Mother. It happened after we had played two games and Kelly had won.

> 'What's next?' asked Mother and Kelly wanted us to get up and form a circle and sing 'A farmer wants a wife . . .'. Kelly said I should stand in the centre, so they sang and I chose her. She was very excited but afterwards Mother said they couldn't continue as they would need many more children, and she should think of something else. Kelly wanted to play mother, father, nanny, and somebody should be the mother. Nobody said anything so, as Kelly asked again and again, Mother said, she was too tired to stand up. Then she gave her another reason, namely, that she had gone to her gymnastic class and she could feel the ache in her legs. Kelly insisted and when she saw she couldn't succeed, she got angry, blaming Mother for spoiling her game and disappeared behind the sofa. Mother tried to calm her and suggested other games but Kelly was cross and didn't want to play anything else.

This sequence shows clearly Mother's limitations in responding to Kelly's feelings and wishes. If we keep in mind that Kelly had spent the whole day with her father, Kelly's wish to play games about a whole family is evidence of her attempt to symbolise her internal situation. But obviously it is too painful for Mother to think about absent parts of the family. Mother seemed to take this game too literally and may have felt accused not only of stopping the play but also of destroying the family. Kelly is quite insistent and does not give up easily. She is flexible enough to modify her proposal but again Mother cannot join in.

What happened when Kelly's feelings were not contained in the observation?

She was offended and angry and went upstairs. Mother followed her after a few minutes and I went after Mother. Mother said she was often like this when she had spent the day with Father. Kelly was in her room lying on her tummy looking angry but not crying. Mother sat down next to her on the bed and tried to explain again, that three women wouldn't like to play 'Father, Mother, Child . . .' and she also referred to me, explaining that I was there to watch her play. I remained close to the door and looked at them. Whatever Mother suggested playing with, the doll's house or kitchen, Kelly said 'No, I don't want to.' Finally Mother changed the subject and asked her what she would like to eat, saying that she was tired and hungry. Kelly accepted Mother's idea of mushroom soup, so Mother went out and left the two of us alone. Kelly got cross with me, first telling me that she didn't want to play anything and then that I should leave. 'Go away!', she shouted with an angry voice.

We see again that Mother is not able to be in touch with Kelly's sadness and vulnerability. Even in this situation, when she is hurt and cross, Mother wants her to play for my sake, so that I could observe her, in other words for somebody else's benefit. Finally, when Mother changes the subject and approaches her on a baby level by offering her mushroom soup, there is a reunion. Mother sees that she has a tired, hungry little girl who needs to get a nice meal and to be looked after. Kelly, on the other hand, is not allowed to show her disappointment and sadness. She seems to realise that Mother cannot put up with her provocative behaviour, therefore she projects her anger into me. I am then the abandoned person who is excluded, like her father, as she is from being with him in imagination. It was a real outburst and a painful rejection for me.

Hypothesis 5: Setting and negotiating rules versus inflexible rules or none

In general, Kelly takes in what Mother tells her. The tone of Mother's voice is soft and friendly. She explains to Kelly why she wants her to do something. For example, when Kelly wants to start drawing, Mother explains to her that she will be going to bed in ten minutes and that there would not be enough time to get all the material out. She offers the option of playing with plasticine instead and also gives her a second choice. Kelly listens carefully and decides to play with plasticine.

Father is also able to stick to rules and to make her understand in a playful way. When Kelly asked him to bring her three sheets of paper without saying 'please', he put his hand to his ear and waited silently. She understood immediately and added laughing a loud 'please, Daddy!' Both parents seem to fulfil her wishes as much as possible and give her a reason if they say no.

Hypothesis 6: Acknowledgement and encouragement versus inhibition of the child's activities

Both parents give Kelly a lot of attention and react to her jokes or stories with laughter or by joining in. She seems to be in tune with Father and Mother. It is a mutual, positive reinforcement. When one parent shows her something, Kelly appreciates it and gives her or him the acknowledgement which makes them feel that they are sensitive parents. In all three observations there was partly a genuine aim to entertain but also a show element. For example, Kelly wanted to sing and dance with Father for me, which they then did. The singing together does seem to be fun for them but also shows a seductive quality in Kelly's behaviour. Father seems to be in touch with the problem that Kelly could get a bit carried away.

In the interview Father gave an example of how much he appreciates her. He said:

> She's very funny, she's an hilarious child. . . . She likes to invent stuff, she likes to invent games, she's very creative and she likes to make up songs. . . . I invent songs sometimes when I'm fooling around, I sort of sing something, instead of saying something, I sing it to her. Yes. (Singing) It's time for bed, now, let's go to bed now. (and then, imitating her voice:) 'OK, Dad, if you want to.'

It is clear how much he appreciates her musical talents. He is amazed that she can even sing intervals.

Hypothesis 7: Good social skills sensitivity versus little social contact

Kelly shows several examples of her highly developed social sensitivity and how she can use it. She is able to establish a relationship with me and is interested in my reactions. When she showed me her book which was called *Titchy*, I asked Mother what 'titchy' meant and she looked at me surprised, impressed that even grown-ups can not know simple things. She also shows a high awareness if she is being used. In the observation with Father he tried to manipulate her. He wanted to offer me a cup of tea but did not do it openly but asked Kelly instead whether she would like one. She said 'No'. I thought this might remind her of being used as a go-between when there was tension between her parents.

Analysis of the interview with the parents

In what way can the parents' narratives help us to clarify the hypotheses about the inner conflict in Kelly between, on the one hand, the good and containing mother that allowed her to develop a stable internal object

(Hypothesis 1) and on the other hand the indications of intrusive potential in Mother to project unresolved conflicts into Kelly (Hypothesis 4).

My first approach to understanding their concept of being a mother or father was to ask them when they had first thought about having a child. Mother answered that she had not thought about it, 'it was an accident.' She had been with Kelly's father for two and a half years and said she knew from the first moment she missed her period that she was pregnant. She always wanted the baby. When she told her partner that the test was positive, she added: 'By the way I'm having the baby, whatever you decide.'

This description conveys several messages on different levels. On the one hand she was happy that she was going to have a baby and never had any doubts about it, but there is also a strong infantile part of her that wants to do it all by herself. Father said he had never thought about having a child because:

> I was not sure whether I was intelligent enough, or capable enough in all the different areas. Being a parent, being a good parent, I didn't actually think that this great responsibility was something that I could discharge well. I thought I would do it less than perfectly . . .

When he heard about it, he was pleased, 'yes, very pleased'. He proposed to her and she accepted. He explained what it meant to him. It was:

> a turning point for me, where I would then have to discipline myself and shape up, because I thought I have to become devoted to the child, and less selfish. More aware of the child's needs.

He is obviously very moved at becoming a father but one wonders why he felt he was not good enough to be a father. His doubts and uncertainty about his qualities and the need to discipline himself show his capacity for concerned reflection.

If we return to the suggestion that Mother might have used Kelly's long breast-feeding as a way of feeling unique and needed, and compare this with her own account, we see quite a correspondence. Mother expressed in the interview how much she liked breast-feeding:

> I always wanted to feed her. I just loved breast-feeding. I mean I really enjoyed it. . . . I had no intention to give it up until she was eighteen months anyway because I think it gives them a good start. . . . And when things started going wrong with James and I, it was like a bond between Kelly and I.

Mother made it clear that her identity depends on being the most important person for her child, providing something nobody else can. She also gives the impression of a narcissistic little girl who is showing off and in competition with men. She also told me that she 'felt absolutely fine about feeding wherever she was, railway stations or in business meetings'.

She seemed to have shown all the world what a wonderful breast-feeding mother she was! I asked her how she weaned Kelly and she described it thus:

> Well, we just sat down one day and I just told her: 'Look Kelly (laughs) . . . I really think, we should stop' . . . it was the au pair coming, I think. . . . And I said: 'We can't have you feeding any more, you're too big now' . . . I said: 'We are going to do it on Monday.' On Monday we just stopped. That was it. And we never looked back.

This really does not sound like a mother–child interaction but rather like a conversation between two people at the same level who decide 'we both have to stop' and then both stick to it. The long breast-feeding, until Kelly was 2 years old, could also be seen as an indicator that Kelly is used as a substitute for a missing sexual relationship. In the interview, both parents confirm this assumption. When I asked Mother about the impact of Kelly on her marriage, she gave a confused answer. Firstly she said: 'I think our relationship would have gone down the pan anyway. When I think back now, things were going wrong before I got pregnant. . . . It was basically the sex thing.' Then she got pregnant, they got married and 'everything looked great'. When she started to work part-time as a teacher she felt she 'had it all: Kelly, my job, my career, my husband, everything looked OK'. 'I stayed with him for as long as I did because of Kelly.' She made it clear that she would have never put up with all this, namely, her husband's violence, if it had just been her. She said:

> He's beaten me a few times, one time my mother was in the house and I hadn't told her about it and she was really really shocked, really frightened for me. And so she stayed here for a while. I had a very brief relationship with somebody else. That's why it all got really difficult. I met him a couple of times and James found out about him. I mean I stopped seeing him. But he didn't believe me. Then he put a tapping device on the phone to tape all my phone calls . . . the day I found it, I thought this man is capable of anything. You know, he's obviously not predictable or safe at all. . . . I wasn't eating . . . I couldn't sleep . . . and I said: 'No, I'm gonna leave' . . . and then on a Friday evening he always went out, so as soon as he'd gone out . . . we just went. I left him a note and explained everything.

So she just disappeared without telling him anything in advance because she was frightened of him.

From Father's perspective, things looked different. He said it was extremely painful for him and he found it difficult to talk about. He then told his version:

> Well, when Katherine was pregnant she was not really well and rejected

me sexually. And we hadn't had sex all the time she was pregnant and we didn't have sex after Kelly was born either. I mean the fact that Katherine rejected me, was not much fun but er, I just accepted it, that's part of the new responsibility . . .

The description of the pregnancy by both parents is consistent. Mother admitted that he was very caring during that time, gave her massage, went with her to ante-natal classes and read a lot of books about birth. He never wanted the divorce because he 'didn't want his child not to be with her father'. He kept referring to this 'painful process'. It was impossible for him to go into any details. He probably felt ashamed of his violence and jealousy.

During all these upheavals both parents were able to keep the fighting away from Kelly and the observer. The observation went on and the observer was not at all aware of the dramatic separation. This shows a mature quality in each of them, that they are able to contain their hatred, disappointment and violence and not to take it out on the child. They both seemed to trust each other in relation to Kelly.

In their attitude towards Kelly both parents show a sense of humanity, kindness and understanding, combined with strictness and a setting of limits, that provide a clear orientation, enabling Kelly to internalise some elements of a good object. On the other hand, one is left concerned about the explosive quality of the conflict between the parents and the collapse of their communication. We can speculate that neither of them was able to be in touch with their own infantile needs and feelings when they were confronted with the new child. Mother might have projected her rivalry into Father and might have pushed him out as though he were a sibling and he might then have acted out the rage and rivalry, literally forcing them back into her in his assaults. Father might have been afraid of his aggressive feelings towards the baby and might have unconsciously protected the baby in Mother's belly by not having sexual intercourse. He made a remark at the end of the interview that 'he always had the fantasy of having sex with a pregnant woman', but the collapse of the sexual relationship at the beginning of the pregnancy indicates that neither had a strong adult self. Their relationship was probably undermined by the unexpected pregnancy and there was no evident reflection as to why he was so upset or why she had to do it all by herself and be the powerful mother. Perhaps there was an infantile neediness in both of them and this may have been the basis of their relationship, interrupted by the arrival of a real baby.

After the divorce, Father took her every morning to the playgroup. I quote a key experience Father mentioned:

After about six months, er, just one day, for no reason at all, we were in the park just feeding the ducks or whatever before we went to the . . .

playgroup and . . . she just ran away and then . . . she just turned round and ran straight back to me and just said: 'Daddy, I love you. I miss you!' And I thought, it is worthwhile. It does work. It does work.

Whether Father can build up a life for himself again, and have another, satisfactory relationship, or concentrate only on Kelly, will have considerable relevance for Kelly's own development.

The remaining hypotheses

I shall briefly discuss my other hypotheses. Father is very proud of her and describes her vividly:

She's good fun and I love the idea that she's really creative . . . at the nursery. She would take the initiative on things and the other kids wouldn't . . . and she'd say: 'Let's do this!' And the others: 'All right', and they'd go and do it. But until she said: 'Let's do it', now they wouldn't have the idea, that's what she's like and she's very kind of positive.

He is sure 'she's her own person' even now when she is so young. These quotations support the hypothesis that Kelly would have quite a dominant position in groups (Hypothesis 7) and make use of her stimulating environment at home (Hypothesis 2). She can influence other children with her imaginative and creative ideas (Hypothesis 5) and she is accepted as a group leader.

Summarising, one could say that the hypothesis of Kelly having developed good internal objects is only partly supported by the narrative of both parents, who emphasise how important she is for them and that they are both identified with her. The over-idealisation and the lack of real concern from Kelly's mother indicates split-off parts of her personality which are not integrated. The idea that Kelly might also have to deal with strong projections seems also confirmed by the material. She might be placed under considerable pressure to take care of both parents: we hear how enormously important she is for Father and that she gives her mother's life a meaning. She had no chance of experiencing the 'threeness' of an Oedipal configuration.

Transgenerational influence

I was led to reflect on how Kelly's mother and father related to their own parents, and what kind of unsolved inner conflicts they might have that could influence Kelly's development. Doing this does not mean I would suggest that there was a causal linear connection. Internal objects cannot be understood as copies of the real relationship to the primary objects, but are always modified and transformed by the child's unconscious phantasies, wishes and impulses. The inner objects consist of different layers. This is a result of the child's relationships first to part objects, a consequence of splitting processes and paranoid anxieties on a deeper level, and later in more integrated form marked by the recognition of Mother and Father as whole persons. Hanna Segal (1973: ix) points out that Melanie Klein's concept of 'position' emphasises the fact that this phenomenon was not simply a passing 'stage' or a 'phase' but 'a specific configuration of object relations, anxieties and defences which persist throughout life'.

The parent's influence on a child cannot be compared with pieces of a puzzle that fit together but the parent's behaviour is something to which the child has to respond. Even if the child pretends or avoids acknowledging painful experiences, this response structures the child's defensive formation. Selma Fraiberg (1980) showed how children with an aggressive and intrusive mother develop a pattern of behaviour which serves the function of regulating negative affects. After a few weeks, the child does not look anxious when it is touched or tossed around roughly but joins in with laughter and excitement. Thus the child wards off painful feelings engendered by the empathic failure of the primary caretaker. Fraiberg shows that babies respond differently to disorganised, depressed or psychotic mothers who are absent-minded and cannot be in tune with the baby's needs and responses. One cannot predict how a particular baby will react, but it has to cope with it in some way. A child with a vigorous constitution can tolerate an absent-minded or intrusive mother better than a more delicate child who might give up more easily and lose a will of its own.

By the same logic we cannot know the reason for a particular behaviour of a child. Piontelli has described in her book *Backwards in Time* (1986) how two children, who both failed to achieve an object relationship which could foster symbol formation, developed in completely different environments. One child, Martin, from a malignant, deprived social background represents a failure in post-natal adjustment whereas Jack, the second observed child, cannot establish a relationship to his warm but somehow emotionally burnt out middle-class mother. Both show the same symptoms of non-autistic infantile psychoses when they move 'backwards in time to an illusory womb-like state' as Piontelli puts it (Piontelli 1986: 11).

Some important studies about this issue of intergenerational psychic process have been done by Peter Fonagy (1994) to link the infant–mother attachment and early manifestations of defence behaviour in infants. The aim of the study is to: 'provide a metapsychological perspective with which to evaluate data concerning the intergenerational concordance in relationship patterns between mother's subjective experience of her own childhood and the quality of the relationship between her and her child' (Fonagy 1994: 1). The data of this research is not collected by infant observation but by the 'Strange Situation Test' and the 'Adult Attachment Interview' (Ainsworth *et al.* 1978).

Here is an example of how the transgenerational pattern emerges. In the interview, Kelly's mother characterised her relationship with her parents with the statement: 'I'll never satisfy my parents.' She went on to say:

> Well, my parents got divorced when I was nine. Before that my father was hardly ever there. He was always working away, and working late. So I didn't have, I didn't see very much of him. But I always adored him and wanted his time. I remember feeling really frustrated because I hardly saw him. My mother was always around. She didn't go back to work until I was about 8. . . . We don't get on that brilliantly now; we're very different.

Mother is critical about her own mother who she felt did not understand her, and she therefore wants to be a different sort of mother. She always had the feeling that she did not get enough from her. She is convinced that she had to take the blame for everything and that her sister, if anyone, was her favourite. Her mother considered life as a struggle and yet now, with Kelly, she is different:

> She spoils her. She never spoiled me, I don't remember her spoiling me . . . she lets Kelly do things she'd never let me do. . . . She's much softer with her than she was with me.

We learn that she left her mother in a way similar to her departure from her husband.

> I left her a note on the bread bin saying: 'Mum, I'm leaving home on Saturday, I can't stand it any more. I know, you wouldn't agree with me, I know you think I can't manage, but I'm going to do it.' She just didn't speak to me. And I just moved out.

Later in the interview, Kelly's mother gives an example of how distorted her perception of Kelly is by projecting her inner critical mother into her. When Kelly complains that she is working too hard, Mother cannot understand it as Kelly's wish to be with her, but sees it as an assault. She also feels attacked and criticised as messy and untidy when Kelly is putting things back in a special place. She gets annoyed when Kelly tells her that things have to go back in the right place. Sometimes she feels she is 'being attacked from both sides'.

Kelly's mother's relationship with her father is more harmonious and seems to be better integrated. She describes him as very loving but not interested in the children, as they 'interrupted his life'. He never spent holidays with them, he was always working, even reading a book at the table at mealtimes, 'he was totally absorbed in himself'. Now he has changed and is much better, more attentive and interested in herself and Kelly. She says,

> He is a different person now ... he sends her clothes and he sends her cards and he speaks to her on the phone and you know, when he comes over he makes a fuss of her and he seems much more relaxed with her than he ever was with us.

Talking in such an understanding and conciliatory way about her own father enables her to see similarities between her former husband and her father. She said, 'he is a lot like my father'. He is also:

> intelligent, well-read and mad about films, mad about music. I mean, he just takes everything in. My dad is the same.

When we hear about her urgent wish to get time and attention from her own father one wonders whether she could have been jealous when Kelly was the centre of interest for her husband.

What is Kelly's father's relationship towards his parents like? He answered the question as follows:

> Well, I'm an only child. My father is dead now, my mother is still alive. I would say that I was extremely fortunate. I had a happy childhood, I was very lucky. I was even aware of my good fortune when I was young, when most kids really aren't.

He continues to describe them as kind, he appreciates their common sense, their care in general. He praises them in many respects:

> They were good parents, they were interested and stimulating parents to have. Interested in lots of things ...

Kelly's father talks about his father as a sensitive man who was at times quite withdrawn and could be very quiet. He was interested in reading and in sport. He seems to admire him and to be identified with him. He gives this characterisation of his mother's personality:

> Well, my mother is another kind of person altogether, very strong. She came from a very poor background, with extreme poverty during the depression. . . . She's very strong, very strong, she has a lot of common sense, a very straight talking sort of a person, very generous and a very important person in my life.

From the material provided, it is not clear why he himself feels so unworthy and damaged. Only when I asked him to compare himself with his parents did he mention a slightly critical view of them:

> They did something which parents of ... only children do tend to do. I

think they were a bit too concerned about things going wrong, a bit too
concerned with a 'what-if' . . .

He connects this 'what if' attitude with his lack of self-esteem, so he is
aware of the impact it had on him.

The picture of Kelly's father remains contradictory. He is positively
identified with Kelly, encourages her interests and takes considerable
pleasure in her development but, on the other hand, he does not want to
recognise any resemblance or similarities between them.

Perception of the observation by the family

Reading the account of the original observation one gets the idea that
there was a strong wish in Mother and later in Kelly to make the observer
a substitute for the almost absent father. This was also the impression of
the observer herself and of the seminar group; she was advised to find an
appropriate distance, keeping a balance between taking up too distant a
position and showing empathy and understanding.

The observer seemed able to resist all attempts to make her a member
of the family and to establish an acceptable position as an observer. Mother
was able to keep the observation going even in this chaotic period of her
life. One might guess that the continuity of the observation was a reliable
support for Mother and Kelly. The rather passive role of observer might
also have inspired the idea of a safe person in contrast to the frightening
husband in Mother's mind. Taking into consideration the observer's rather
quiet personality, there seems to be a fit between her style, her personality
and the need of the family for her to be like this. She may indeed have
picked up in her counter-transference the gentle, low-key kind of approach
needed to ease the stressful situation.

In the follow-up observations Kelly was able to establish a strong
relationship with me as an observer. I was struck by the way she and her
parents could link up my follow-up observation with the earlier two-year
observation.

When I asked the parents in the interview how they experienced the
observation, both of them described Kelly as having a similar reaction to
their own. Mother thought Kelly 'found it quite strange because she didn't
interact very much'. She quoted Kelly who had referred to the observer
as 'that one who wants to watch me'. Asked about her own expectations,
Mother clearly said that she had thought the observer would be more
involved with the child as she grew older, but also more available to her,
'company' for her. She expressed her disappointment when she said: 'I
felt a bit like a showcase sometimes.' The fact that she was 'fond of her',
as she put it, 'and really got on fine with her' might have made it even
more disappointing for her. As this was also the time when her marriage

was deteriorating, one is inclined to think that Mother might have hoped for some emotional compensation from the observer.

Father met the observer during the two years only on three or four occasions during observations. Father felt it was a bit strange and then came to terms with it once the observer had explained to him 'that she was training herself to be observant'. Father could also express his wish to hear something about Kelly but understood that the observer couldn't talk to him because he was concentrating on Kelly. There seemed to be an identification between Father and observer when he gave a vivid description of how he did a night school course in photography 'that made me look more closely at things'. He found himself observing the body language of his friend's children and of his daughter. Father described Kelly's reaction to the observer as much like his own. He said:

> She just accepted she was only observing her. . . . I think once that she realised that there was no conversation or games with her, that she just sort of thought, oh she is there and she doesn't talk to me and that's OK.

Conclusion

I would now like to draw some conclusions about my two main questions, namely, the validity of infant observation as a method and second, what was learned about Kelly's development and the transgenerational pattern in this case study.

In reading the original paper about Kelly's development I gained a clear picture of her personality. But I was struck and indeed amazed that the observer had had so little awareness of the marriage difficulties and did not know about the outbursts of violence.

Reflections on methodology

The idea of using the same observation method in the follow-up study proved to be fruitful. It also demonstrated the emotional significance of the observer since the relationship between her and the family was strong enough to be linked with a new person doing the follow-up study. My visit did not feel like a first observation; there was mutual trust and openness as if we had known each other for a long time. I had expected that I would be influenced by my knowledge of the written account of the first observation and the way the observer had described the interaction in the family, but I found myself fully concentrating on the here-and-now, receptive to the particular situation and events to which I was exposed.

The predictions which derived from the first observation were discussed with the observer and she then provided additional material. The central dilemma of a psychoanalytically oriented observation is that one has to draw conclusions from the observed behaviour about the inner world of the child, her characteristic anxieties, defences and mental structure. The two observations, however, showed a convincing consistency in the quality of interactions in the family.

The interview with both the parents provides new material about their understanding of themselves as parents, modelled on recollections of their own parents. Their description of Kelly's reaction to the observer shows how much they tended to project their own feelings into Kelly. Mother felt partly neglected and 'used' and could express her wish to get more of the observer's attention. The observer could keep her role as such and her regular visits might even have provided some stability throughout the time of separation. The interview also reveals the limitations of the observation, where important background information is missing.

Themes in Kelly's development

When we compare the material from the follow-up observation and the interviews with the first hypothesis, the picture of Kelly changed in some respects. The impression of Kelly's development was more optimistic after the first two years, whereas her situation seems to be more precarious two years later. We assumed that Kelly had internalised a good primary object, which would enable her to cope with problems and that therefore she would develop good self-esteem. Also, that the safe and stimulating environment would facilitate her ability to symbolise and express herself in a creative way. Two years later, we see a little schoolgirl who loves to learn, is proud of her achievements, and spontaneously shows her books and how well she can read to the observer. She is creative in elaborating games, she can express herself verbally very well, tells stories to her dolls and sings her own songs. One can say that in several areas she has fulfilled the predictions. She also has a lot of physical contact with her parents, indicating a trusting relationship with them. However, she seems to have little space to express negative or aggressive feelings when she is with her mother. Kelly has to be reasonable and understanding, and is not allowed to complain about her mother's planned departure the next day. So one wonders whether she really had an opportunity to integrate positive and negative feelings, an experience that leads to a sense of wholeness.

When we look at her level of anxiety and Mother's ability to contain her anxieties, we see clear limitations in Mother. As a baby, Kelly was quite uncontrollable in her distress about the absent mother, and the prolonged breast-feeding up to the age of 2 made us wonder about compensating instead of accepting the loss via a mourning process. Later on, when Kelly is described as an actress, playing for rewarding laughs and smiles, we suggested a tendency to cover deeper feelings, loss and separation, behind a manic hyperactivity. In the follow-up observation we can clearly see Mother's limitations in containing Kelly's wish for a family all together, her symbolised wish for Father's presence. Both parents over-idealise Kelly and give her a central role in their lives. This could be a burden for her, to show only the sunny side of her personality in order not to disappoint them. There is a sense of alarm about Mother's distorted perception of Kelly, when she interprets Kelly's wish to put things back as criticising and controlling her. A mother who feels 'attacked from both sides', Mother projects her own critical mother into Kelly. Furthermore, we do not know what impact the violence of her father has had on Kelly.

When Kelly's anxiety and frustration are not contained by Mother but pushed back into her, Kelly projects it into the observer. I am then the abandoned person who should leave – quite a powerful form of 'acting out'. Therefore, we will have to reformulate the assumption of a good internal object, as there seem to be persecutory aspects that are external-ised. The idealisation by the parents might contribute to the development of a 'false self' as Winnicott (1965) called it, to be the Kelly her parents expect her to be, disconnected from her darker feelings.

With respect to the dimensions of parental behaviour, for example, how they set rules and negotiate them, and also how they acknowledge Kelly's abilities and activities, the two observations are quite consistent. Both parents are able to set limits, explaining why they have to say no. They do not humiliate Kelly but give her time to think over and make sugges-tions about how to solve a problem. They provide a stimulating environment with games, creative play, music and drawing. They both enjoy her creative activities. There might be a danger of becoming a little princess when everything she does is so important to them. Her good sense of humour and her generosity of mind make her a popular member of the group; she will probably be a group leader and the centre of attention.

In summary, we would say that it is striking how well Kelly is developing despite the dramatic separation of her parents; Kelly shows a clear capacity to keep both households in her mind. However, the strong pressure on her to be special, combined with the lack of containment of her anxieties, will make integration more difficult. She may well have problems in forming stable relationships in the future.

ACKNOWLEDGEMENTS

The research was made possible by a fellowship from the Austrian 'Fonds zur Förderung der wissenschaftlichen Forschung'.

I would like to particularly thank Margaret Rustin for her help and support throughout the project, and Elizabeth Bradley, Hélène Dubinsky,

Anton Obholzer, David Trevatt and Isca Wittenberg for their support and encouragement.

REFERENCES

Ainsworth, M., Blehar, M. C., Waters, E. and Wall, S. (1978) *Patterns of Attachment: A Psychological Study of the Strange Situation*, Hillsdale, NJ.: Lawrence Erlbaun.

Alvarez, A. (1992) *Live Company. Psychoanalytic Psychotherapy with Autistic, Borderline, Deprived and Abused Children*, London: Tavistock/Routledge.

Coolican, H. (1970) *Research Methods and Statistics in Psychology*, London: Hodder and Stoughton Educational.

Fonagy, P. (1994) 'The integration of psychoanalytic theory and work on attachment: the issue of intergenerational psychic processes', in *Psychoanalysis and Development. Representations and Narratives*, New York: New York University Press.

Fraiberg, S. (1980) *Clinical Studies in Infant Mental Health. The First year of Life*, London Tavistock Publications.

Freud, S. (1905) *Three Essays on Sexuality, Standard Edition* 7, London: Hogarth Press.

Piontelli, A. (1986) *Backwards in Time, A Study in Infant Observation by the Method of Esther Bick*, Strath Tay, Perthshire: Clunie Press.

Thomas, A. and Chess, S. (1977) *Temperament and Development*, New York: Brunner/Mazel.

Segal, H. (1973) *Introduction to the Work of Melanie Klein*, London: Karnac Books.

Waddell, M. (1994) *The Teenage Years. Understanding 12–14 Year Olds*, London: Rosendale Press.

Winnicott, D. W. (1965) 'Ego distortion in terms of true and false self', in *The Maturational Process and the Facilitating Environment*, London: Hogarth Press (first published 1960).

Chapter 12

Observing when infants are at potential risk

Reflections from a study of five infants, concentrating on observations of a Bengali infant

Stephen Briggs

This chapter describes some of the work undertaken as part of a research project. The aim was to observe a small sample of infants at potential risk, and to see what this could tell us, first, about the development of infants in these circumstances, and second, about the role of observation as a research tool.

I therefore observed five infants weekly, from birth to 2 years, a process involving some 400 individual observations. The five infants were selected through contacting a range of referral sources: health visitors, social workers, and a psychotherapist, who were known to be involved with populations of 'at risk' children and their families. Risk was not discussed with the referrers or families before observations in order not to skew the data. Initial discussions were carefully recorded and an assessment of risk made on the basis of this. I expected to be confronted with problems relating to the emotional development of the infants, and the boundary between these problems and physical hurting of the infants.

The sample came from a range of social class and cultural backgrounds, including a white English working-class family, a single parent, a Bengali family and a white diplomatic family from an English-speaking country. The infants observed were two girls and three boys; one was a firstborn and the others ranged from second to ninth in the family.

Observing five infants simultaneously afforded me the opportunity of observing the features and qualities of the development of each infant and also the possibility of making comparisons. The naturalistic method of infant observation gives very detailed information about the development of any one infant but it does not provide explicit means of making comparison. The task of comparison involved me in extensive work of a methodological nature, and I have given detailed accounts of this elsewhere (Briggs 1996, 1997). From this work, in general terms, there emerged several fruitful areas of a comparative nature. Of particular relevance for the study of infants at risk was the operationalisation of Bion's theory of the role of mother's 'reverie' (Bion 1962). Reverie comprises a state of mind in the mother (or parent) in which she allows the baby's experiences to enter her mind, so that she can think about and gather a sense of the meaning of these infantile communications. These are then used to formulate, consciously and unconsciously, responses to the infant's communications and needs. The baby experiences containment from the mother's emotional work of first allowing the infant's experiences to permeate her, making sense of these communications before responding to the baby, through her words, gestures and deeds, and thus conveying her understanding of his needs.

In this sample of five infants, where I was observing infants in a range of stressful circumstances, it was important to take into account the mothers' states of mind and the impact of these on the babies, and also, of equal importance, the infants' responses. Within my sample there was a considerable difference observed between the different babies' capacities to deal with situations. What became clear was the importance for each infant of the adaptive, or defensive, measures they developed alongside the capacity to sustain an interest in relationships both in the outside world and their own emerging internal worlds.

In my exploration of the quality of containment available to each of the infants in my study I have attempted to describe, using an image of shape, how the quality of receptivity in the parents in interaction with the infants shifts from Bion's idea of reverie (concave) to parenting where the infantile communication is missed or blocked (flat) to that where the parent activity actively intrudes upon the infant (convex). Such intrusions can be primarily emotional intrusions of the parents' own uncontained, distressing or disturbing experiences and they can be physical intrusions. Both the flat unresponsive emotional states and the intrusive, convex states can precipitate 'at risk' situations for the infant.

What made the task of analysis of the observer–observed relationship so difficult in this sample of infants is that the problems encountered by all the infants in the sample, at least through parts of the observation, were so acute that, in the interests of concern for their welfare and development, I was obliged to adopt a more interventionist approach to observation than is traditionally assumed. The material generated by the observations of the infants in this sample of 'at risk' infants illustrates the 'containing' function performed by any observer in the task of 'observing' an infant.

THE FAMILY

In order to illustrate the processes of observing an infant at potential risk, and to demonstrate the kind of material that emerged in this study, I shall focus in this chapter on one of the five infants in the sample. I shall call him Hashmat. This was a most complex observation to undertake and think about. He was the ninth boy in a Bengali family whose parents spoke very little English, and who adhered strongly to a traditional way of life. The family size, the cultural difference between the family and the observer, and the fact that there was little common ground in terms of verbal communication created an unusual observational context. As observer I found it necessary to suspend judgement; the task of contending with ambiguous communication was powerfully present.

I was introduced to the family through a health visitor, whose comments to me suggested that she had no particular concerns about this baby, nor about the family as a whole; no other child in the family had caused particular problems, nor had there been stillbirths, infant deaths, etc. Therefore, although risk was not identified by the referral source, the circumstances of the family suggested to me that it would be worthwhile to go ahead with the observation.

I was taken to meet the family – by appointment – by the health visitor and an interpreter. I was told that neither parent spoke much English, but that the father was the more fluent of the two. The family live in a four-bedroom flat on a large estate which is almost totally Bengali. In this part of London there is a community of some 40,000 Bengali. The pattern of Bengali migration is poorly documented, though Watson (1977) describes the experiences of Bengali males and in particular their separations from and reunions with their families. The main migration occurred after the war with Pakistan, though many, like Hashmat's father, came to this country much earlier, in 1960.

Their flat I described at the time as 'cavernous'; a long corridor off which there were bedrooms led to a warm living room. Javed Ahmed, the father, spoke in Bengali through the interpreter, impressing on us his role. His wife Rani waited until permission was given to sit down, and father spoke about his wife's view of the observation. Javed was quite portly, about 50, with a damaged eye. He did not work outside the home and throughout was a significant presence in observations. Rani was darker skinned, with a warm smile and looked younger than her husband – under 40 I guessed. Both were traditionally dressed and Rani's pregnancy showed very little. I wondered how I could obtain the mother's view of the observation and asked, through the interpreter and Javed how they would feel about my observing, especially when mother was feeding the baby. Javed replied that his wife would not breast-feed. She had tried with the older children but did not have enough milk and she would bottle-feed the new baby. He spoke to his wife who nodded and smiled at me.

I felt clear that the parents had agreed to the observation, and appeared to welcome the interest in their family. I was also sure their motivation was more complex than this and wondered what I might represent, or come to represent for them. I also wondered how I might be able to understand, and try to avoid misunderstanding, their communications. The potential for misunderstanding became apparent when the health visitor contacted me two months ahead of the time of the expected birth date, to announce that the baby was born. She was somewhat surprised but told me the baby was full-term. 'They must have got their dates wrong', she added, and thus conveyed a sense of frustration – as though the family had made her feel incompetent. This was the first of a number of key events that occurred in my association with this family, where the element of total surprise, lack of preparation or of communication about the event were features, raising the ambiguous issue of the quality of communications between white professionals and the family; who did not understand whom? Or did the family not know themselves?

It soon became apparent that it would be difficult to describe the quality of containment for Hashmat, within a family Gestalt where each member had a role and function in terms of parenting the infant. In order to think about the kind of containment experienced by Hashmat, it was important to take into account the contribution of the family members as a unit, as well as quality of containment provided by Hashmat's mother. Three distinct and different family patterns were observed at different times during the observations.

First, and most prevalent was a 'group' culture, where the primary notion was that any family member could look after the baby as well as anyone else. As the observer I was initially invited to join this shared phantasy, being asked to feed Hashmat, hold him and to be similarly involved with the other children. Parental functions were delegated to different family members. However, at other times the siblings would attack the infant, either – more usually – physically hurting the baby, or – more rarely – inflicting some emotionally cruel situation upon him. Mother's approach was characterised by, first, not thinking, not noticing or passing the baby to someone else (flat), and father's by attempts at authoritarianism; cracking the whip (convex). It was of interest why parental authority was absent when parents were physically absent. At these times, the notion of a protecting parent, held in the mind by the child, was also absent. The siblings joined together to gang up on the baby. At such times Hashmat was actually at risk and on occasions I was forced to drop the more conventional observer role and actively intervene to physically protect either Hashmat or one of the younger children.

Second, by way of contrast, there were passages of time where, with most of the older boys out of the house, the family, with both mother and father at home, resembled much more a nuclear family, where individual attention was possible. In contrast to the first pattern of relating, these passages seemed extremely peaceful, and included interaction between parents and infant. In these periods mother was occasionally capable of a vigorous containment, although she seldom demonstrated this capacity. For large parts of the observation she was much more passive than this, undeniably depressed and dealing with the very great burden of her situation by not thinking, and through escape into a phantasy world. For example, she was completely captivated by a video of an Asian woman as heroine, the portrayal of whom was as far from her actual situation as could possibly be imagined. On other occasions, when she allowed herself to think, especially about the dependency needs of her children, she became very easily overwhelmed, and portrayed real helplessness. In the second year, when I was more actively involved with Hashmat, she was at times more responsive and able to observe his behaviour and interactions with me with some interest.

Father was to an extent supportive in this second 'mode' of parenting. Tasks were divided between them; he dealt with the outside – shopping, collecting children from school. She prepared the food and fed the children. Father would hold the infant, smile at him, sing a soothing lullaby to him.

Third, though this was seen much less often, there were periods of time when the adults outnumbered the children, namely, when mother's mother, other relatives and friends were present. These events produced different reactions in terms of the quality of the containing environment. When mother's own mother was present there appeared to be a more vigorous approach not only to the children but also to the quality of communication. Mother on these occasions found the wherewithal to speak clearly in English. It was also, paradoxically, when other adults were present that the family – and particularly the parents – moved into a most 'switched off' mode of functioning, where the children were left literally to attend to themselves. For example, when Hashmat was sixteen weeks, both he and Shakil were left to cry without being attended to, as mother was involved in a kind of ritualistic food preparation, imbued with sensuality.

Another important dimension to the observation of this particular family was the history of events as they unfolded during the observational period. Most notably I observed the arrival of two babies (Hashmat and his younger brother Fashmat, born just before Hashmat's first birthday). During Hashmat's second year, the Bangladesh cyclone took many lives and this was followed by father's visit there. One of the older boys told me that 'Bangladesh is slipping into the sea'. This is then an uprooted family with a relationship to another country, Bangladesh. Probably pertinent here is the impact of previous history; Javed's parents had died in Bangladesh whilst he lived in England (but before the observations started). He may have lost relatives in the cyclone. In the immediate environment I heard from time to time – from inside the family and outside sources – of race-fuelled conflicts. During the observational period the older boys were leaving school and starting work. Four of them were wage earners before the end of the observation. All of these events I heard about in passing; a child would mention something to me – for example, that the oldest boy now lived away from home. Often the impact of events was gleaned from the experience of observing before the event was named. Naming of things was not a family forte. The task of naming things rested with the eight-year-old, a benign soft-featured boy who had the capacity to give names to feelings, on behalf of the family. I shall refer to his part later.

THE OBSERVATIONAL ROLE

Communication between myself and Hashmat's parents took place very concretely; there were few and limited verbal exchanges. Actions became important communications, and through these a particular mode of relating was established, through experience, in which I was able to negotiate a position where the main observing function, attention, particularly to the emotional communications of the infant, was maintained. It was also important to find ways of responding appropriately to events, within the matrix of the parents' spoken and unspoken expectations of the observer and in response to Hashmat's communications to me. Not to have responded in these ways would have been either unethical or dangerous or amounting to a perturbation (Murray and Trevarthen 1986). The role of the observer therefore became a combination of an observer/parent figure, or 'auxiliary parent'. The role had specific functions for the development of the infant Hashmat. These were, first, that of enabling him to share some emotional states, and second of providing a focus where thinking enabled him to maintain contact between different aspects of himself. A complex relationship therefore developed between Hashmat and myself which included, especially in his second year, communication to me of his emotional states and a curiosity about me and my role. His play in my presence was rich and evocative of his most important preoccupations and concerns. In my study as a whole, I found that patterns of relationship between myself and infants and their parents developed, either along the lines seen here, of the role of 'auxiliary parent' or where the role was more primarily concerned with supporting the parent, as a 'parental container'. The implications are that the qualities of attentiveness and mindfulness in an observer can support a more resilient development in infancy. The role may be developed in a way in which professionals can use it to make accurate, informed interventions in families.

THE FIRST THREE MONTHS: THE CONTAINING ENVIRONMENT

At the beginning of the observations I was given a concrete expression of the culture of the family and the parents' views of my role of observer. Father prayed in front of me, and I was offered curry and rice. Then father showed me the baby by offering him to me to hold. I was thus introduced to Hashmat, nine days old, an unnamed baby dressed in a pink babygro:

> I saw the baby under a pile of blankets in the corner of the room, a snuffling sound alerting me to his presence. Both father Javed and mother Rani came into the room and the baby cried a little. Javed picked him up and held him out to show me. He offered him to me to hold, and he put him on my lap. Baby screwed up his eyes and cried. He has a shock of dark hair, pale fingers, and seemed delicate, but full-term. I asked mother if she wanted to take him as he continued to cry, and she did so, holding him, then sitting down on the sofa. Baby stopped crying and Rani asked father to pass the bottle, and she gave the bottle, cradling baby on her right arm, her large hand held out open palmed. Hashmat took the bottle and sucked, closing his eyes. Rani looked at him and then at me, smiling a little self-consciously.

The pattern where Hashmat maintained eye or mouth contact with mother, but not both, continued. It became a feature, whereby the idea that there was no eye contact between them seemed to be jointly accepted. This way of feeding was so regularly repeated that it held the quality of a sculpt. For example, when Hashmat was nine weeks:

> Rani looked up and smiled and continued to feed Hashmat. She held him loosely, watching television, her large hand open and then just touching his arm. His eyes were open and looking also in the direction of the television. He sucked quietly.

Mother and infant together accommodated to this pattern of relating to each other; the accommodation in the 'fit' between mother and infant had them turning towards a third person or object. The emotional contact in feeding lay outside the mother–infant couple, in the 'group', the father, one of the eight brothers, the television and me, the observer. Here there were a wide range of objects of different qualities. The television, in this example, had a mindless quality. Father contributed a well-meaning but usually noisy and intrusive presence. Shakil, the 3-year-old, was noisily attacking, particularly when supported by the older 5-year-old Chalaak. In the observation at nine weeks, for example, Shakil climbed on to the coffee table, prompting father to shout to him to get down. Then:

> Hashmat seemed to splutter over his milk and mother tried to keep the bottle in his mouth, but he continued to splutter and she took it out and seemed to grapple with him, pulling his legs and then sitting him up and patting his back firmly, then putting him over her shoulder and patting him, still firmly. Hashmat continued to cry and struggle, his hands and legs pushing against her, and she seemed to hold him tight.

> He kept crying and she put him down on the sofa, where he kept crying and she spoke to him, soothingly, saying 'alla, alla'.

Mother seemed slow to respond to Hashmat's spluttering and appeared to insist he took the bottle. His protest was quite vigorous, communicating the indigestibility of the experience for him, apparently precipitated by father's shouting. Mother seemed to insist he continued to feed regardless of the interruption, suggesting his emotional responses to the impingements of others in his world were not uppermost in her mind. Mother reported Hashmat not to be feeding well and to be regurgitating feeds. It was not surprising that he vomited so much, as 'indigestible' experiences were present from a number of sources and went unremarked by mother, who left Hashmat to deal with them.

During these first three months I observed both parents relating to Hashmat in different but quite definable modes. Father alternated between holding the baby, singing to him soothingly and moving around the home in a noisily intrusive but apparently unthinking way. Mother presented herself as attentive and responsive at times to his physical needs, but held the baby somewhat loosely, as in the above examples, reflecting the limits of her emotional availability for Hashmat. This was linked with her wish to use me, again concretely, to help with the baby, as indeed the older siblings were employed. When Hashmat was seven weeks she asked me, through one of the older boys, to feed him.

> Rani came into the room where Hashmat, three of the brothers and I were. She carried a bottle. She looked at me and spoke to Miral, who is 14. Miral, translating, said that Hashmat has been vomiting when feeding. I murmured sympathetically, and Miral went on to say that his mother would like me to try feeding him. He passed me the baby and mother passed a shawl. I held him on my lap and Miral went out, returning with two tissues, to catch the expected vomit.

Whilst this presented me with a difficulty, in role as observer, it also evoked father's earlier comment that Rani had insufficient milk herself to feed the children. Overstretched with the demands of nine children, perhaps disappointed that this ninth baby was another boy, mother seemed to wish to delegate the role of feeding, in the face of the difficulties she had reported, to me. At the same time she conveyed that my presence was required in order to help her in her parenting. Later in this observation she demonstrated, concretely, that she was not available, at that time, for Hashmat either emotionally or physically:

> [I was again holding Hashmat] and I stood up as mother reappeared. I showed Hashmat to her and passed him to her. She held out her hands, palms up to prevent me giving her the baby, and gestured to Miral that he should take him.

Mother's unavailability was linked with the position, quite clearly derived from necessity, that the siblings should take an active role in holding, feeding and responding to the baby. By extension, she saw me as part of that group, and this had to be taken into consideration when, as happened frequently, I was left alone in the room with Hashmat and his brothers, causing me to review my observer role again. It was in these circumstances that the unavailability of parental care for Hashmat spilled into something more actively, physically hazardous for Hashmat. An example of this comes from the same observation at seven weeks, when play between the siblings, Miral, Chalaak, who is 5, and Shakil, who is 3, nearly results in Hashmat being injured:

> Hashmat began to cry. Wearily, Miral went over to the cot and lifted him out, holding him in his arms, but continuing to play his wrestling game with Chalaak. Chalaak swung with his leg just missing Hashmat's face, and Shakil got Miral round the middle nearly toppling him and the baby. Hashmat stared wide eyed away from them, his head on one side.

Hashmat was here almost an invisible, incidental presence to the boys in their aggressive games. The murderous intent was verbalised by Shakil when Hashmat was eight weeks:

> Shakil started playing with a football. He said, with menace, 'No baby', and Hashmat lay with his eyes very slightly open as if peering or pretending to be asleep.

When he was twelve weeks he was attacked in a more chilling way by the combination of Shakil and Chalaak:

> With his fingers Chalaak started poking Hashmat's face, rubbing his finger down his cheek. He then got hold of his bib and twisted it with the effect of twisting as if to throttle him. I looked at Chalaak and he stopped. He got off the sofa and started to play his violent game with the other two boys and then Shakil came next to Chalaak on the sofa and grabbed both Hashmat's legs. He started to pull the legs towards him. I said 'No' to Shakil. Hashmat started to cry loudly and persistently. Shakil held on to Hashmat's legs, looking very angrily at me, as I leaned over Hashmat while Shakil swore at me a couple of times. I picked up Hashmat as he continued to cry and held him on my lap. His head went back and he cried, looking at me with a frightened look in his eyes. The boys opened the door and ran out.

Parental absence on these occasions led to the adaptation of my role, and I acted as a parent rather than an observer; it appeared that to have denied this, or to have rigidly maintained a non-interventionist strategy would be incomprehensible within this group style of parenting, and possibly unethical. Some specific and clearly oriented interventions became part of my role.

There was a constant theme of the lack of mediation of emotional experiences within the family or even an acknowledgement of them. Hashmat's siblings were allowed in this way to give expression to their feelings which had as a common element, as graphically verbalised by Shakil, the idea there should be 'no baby'.

THE FIRST THREE MONTHS: HASHMAT'S DEVELOPMENT

Hashmat's response to early experiences within this environment is to become quite withdrawn, peering at the world through closed, or nearly closed eyes, appearing frozen, a frightened animal in a threatening world, showing signs of alertness through barely perceptible movements. He did not grow; he was not thriving. The experiences of assault on his bodily integrity, through noisy intrusion, attacks on his existence by siblings and the lack of emotional space for him in mother's mind, led me to question how he held himself together. He was not a muscular infant, in the way described by Bick (1968), though I did notice on occasions he arched his back and stiffened, flapped his legs and arms, which suggested he was experiencing an unintegrated state. What emerged in the observational material was evidence of a complex relationship between his hand, himself and other people. The development of these relationships can be shown in the context of the quality of parental response to his communications, in sequences from the observations. First, in the observation at nine weeks, when Hashmat spluttered over his milk and father shouted at Shakil to get down from the coffee table, mother grappled and pulled Hashmat and the impact upon me was a powerful one, so much so that I started to feel sick. Then mother spoke soothingly to Hashmat and the observation continued:

> Mother stood up, moving away from him and he quietened. She walked out and Hashmat quietly now flapped his arms and kicked his legs. Shakil then came towards Hashmat, who, with a slight turn of the head, watched him. Shakil came nearer and then touched Hashmat's hand. He leaned over Hashmat and spoke to him, quite loudly. Hashmat gripped Shakil's finger.

Mother seemed unaware of a cause for the spluttering and so could not help Hashmat to find a way through an unpleasant experience. Hashmat did then make a grip with his hand on the available Shakil. Then, when he was eleven weeks, he was asleep and his hand made contact with the blanket under which he was lying:

> As I watched Hashmat, his hands touched one another so that the right

one was resting on the left wrist. He was still for a time until he brought his right hand up and over his head; then he took it down and it caught the lip of the blanket. He shuffled this across his mouth. He twitched his head, eyes closed, from side to side and then cried. He cried once and was quiet, and neither mother nor father reacted. Hashmat resumed sleeping with his hand on the left wrist. Then he repeated his movements, his right leg moving under the blanket, his right hand moving towards his face but catching the blanket which he seemed to pull against his chin uncomfortably. He began to cry, his mouth wide and his hands shaking a little against the blanket. He cried once, and then again, then continuously.

In this sequence, the use of his hand, even whilst he was asleep suggested it helped him provide the contact through which he could develop a phantasy or dream. He also made gestures with his hands which conveyed a clear meaning; for example, his hands came over his eyes as if to shield them. The observation continued:

Hashmat cried, and there was something pitiful in his cries, as though he did not expect a response. He seemed to manage to get his hands to touch each other, but he continued to cry. Mother looked round, while still feeding Shakil, and she smiled at Hashmat. She turned towards the table and took the dinner things out into the kitchen. Hashmat stopped crying and went back to sleep. He lay still and put his right arm across his face as if to shield his eyes. Mother smiled at me as she sat down on the sofa next to Hashmat and took the small blanket behind his head away. She put the bottle to his lips and twisted it until he took it between his lips. He started to suck, quite hungrily, while mother sat looking towards him, but not touching him. He seemed to have his eyes closed, either shut or only very slightly open.

Again at the end of this sequence mother fed Hashmat by routine rather than by his request, and at some distance from him. He did take the bottle, even though it was forced into his mouth. Again the separation of mouth and eye contact with mother was noticeable. His cries earlier in the sequence conveyed a sense that he would not be responded to, overtly being left to cry or, more subjectively, not having his distress mediated through understanding parental responses. He did, however, struggle to relate to others, and his use of his hand is prominent in his repertoire.

The hand grip was developing strongly with variety. It showed he had at least a notion of an object which could hold another, in a three-dimensional way, one containing another. These quiet gestures permitted some psychic survival in the face of a mother who was clearly overwhelmed, and a family setting which was dangerously intrusive. Those hand grips also formed prototypes of relationships which were seen throughout the observations.

In these early observations, I was struck by the contrast between the vulnerable Hashmat, whose development was so delayed, and the rumbustious pair of Shakil and Chalaak. Shakil had at times the attributes of a gangster; Chalaak was the epitome of toughness. Was Hashmat one boy too many in this family, or was there a family pattern whereby survival in a particular way – namely of developing a tough, fighting skin, was part of the culture of development?

DEVELOPMENT FROM THREE MONTHS TO A YEAR

Between three months and a year, Hashmat's behaviour was characterised by sudden spurts of development, which countered the feeling – and fact – that his development was markedly backward. He continued to seem, in his development and relationships with others, to be unadventurous. He was not sitting unaided until eight months and then he began to attempt crawling after nine months. In fact development occurred, as it were, from the outside. Parents put him in a bouncing chair, and later a baby walker, though he had shown no movement towards sitting up, raising his head, or trying to move about. But there were grounds for optimism. At fourteen weeks I saw him for the first time sitting in a baby walker. This elevation was accompanied by a greater sense of curiosity. His hand grip was still evident:

> He looked alertly around the room and in my direction, his hair shaved and his very dark eyes looking out. His legs kicked a little and his arms moved also, his hands touching each other.

Mother was more vigorous in this period. Later in this observation she offered a soothing response when changing Hashmat:

> Hashmat quietened down as soon as Rani started to stroke his legs and bottom with the cotton wool. She cleaned him very thoroughly, quite vigorously at times and then she seemed to clean him with quite smooth movements with the cotton wool, all in her usual unhurried slightly slow way.

Her attention to his skin appeared to give him a sense of his boundaries, of himself. He greeted me with a smile when I arrived for observations, he sought me with his eyes, and there developed a considerable interaction in the relationship with me. It was particularly notable that this relationship hinged around a particular kind of grip, often with the use of the hand, and accompanied by his making sounds. For example at four months two weeks:

Rani rubbed his back more, and then she picked him up and put him in the bouncing chair, and went out, and Hashmat made his high-pitched noises with Shakil riding his bike around. Hashmat seemed about to cry and I leaned forwards and touched his foot and his hand reached down so I put my finger in his hand and he held on to it tightly and pulled my hand towards him and he made noises ranging between content, accompanied by a suggestion of a smile, to distress.

I acknowledged his solitary struggle towards relating inner states. Attempts at language and sharing a wide range of emotions followed. This willingness to communicate continued. When he was six months three weeks:

Hashmat sat and looked at me with a long look. His eyes focused on me steadily, with his face on the brink of tears. His hands moved on the table and he had a small, hard plastic whistle which he held. He cast his eyes in the direction of the door where Rani had gone out. I smiled at him and felt there was something very delicate in his mood, so he could easily shift from smiling to crying. The look he was giving me was held on a gossamer thread. He made a little shrieking noise and I made a soothing one back. He put his finger in his mouth, and he poked with it behind his top gum, his mouth wide open. He took his finger out and dropped the toy whistle over the side. I retrieved it and he looked surprised to see it again, and then he held it.

He seemed to be communicating to me something about his teeth, to be saying 'It hurts'. There followed a weekly ritual where he made lip-smacking gestures to me, which I imitated. His communication of pain was also seen when he was nine months two weeks. Here the communication indicated the nature of the source of his distress:

[He was trying to crawl, but gets his leg caught.] He cried a little and then gently banged his head on the floor some few times. [Father then picked him up and after comforting him passed him to me.] He was hesitant and then touched my hand, grasping my finger, holding it quite tightly. He reached out to me and poked his finger into my mouth . . . He leaned against my chest and banged his head against it, lightly but with a feeling of wanting to make a space there.

Throughout the observation Hashmat had experienced his mother as meta-phorically pregnant, that is, preoccupied with concerns of her own and not open to his needs. Yet there was further evidence when he was ten months seventeen days that Hashmat may be reacting to a real pregnancy:-

Hashmat crawled under the table near Rani's feet, his head nearly touching the underside of the table top. There was no room for him to move unless he dropped down. He seemed to get stuck, and became motionless, frozen, unable to move. Rani's mother leaned down and gently pulled him out backwards, while Rani guided his head to stop it bumping the table.

This sequence brought to my mind the idea of a forceps delivery, with Hashmat playing the baby and his grandmother the midwife. The birth of Fashmat, a few days before Hashmat's first birthday, was one of the most peculiar events in the history of this observation. This was partly because whilst Hashmat seemed in tune with his mother's pregnancy I had failed to spot it! Partly, too, it was because of the family's reaction to it. Father announced the birth in this way:

> Javed Ahmed came in and sat at the table and began to peel an onion with the curved knife. Then he said he may have to go to the hospital and added that his wife had a baby yesterday at 2.30 p.m.; another boy. He was looking pleased, a smile on his face as he spoke to me. Then he carried on peeling the onion.

Meanwhile, the children – Chalaak, Miral and Belal (who is 10) played a game of twenty-four counting fruit:

> Belal said: 'apples, bananas, grapes, pears', and Miral added: 'apples, oranges, grapes, bananas, grapes', to which Belal rejoined, with giggles: 'apples, oranges, grapes, pears, bananas, melon, grapes'.

As the list grew longer and in random style, with repetition, one had the inescapable feeling that they were counting babies! Humour turned to violence at the hands of Siral, the 15-year-old. In the following observation, in the absence of his parents, he enacted the mindless rage against the family's babies, with Hashmat as victim:

> Hashmat, sitting on the windowsill seemed to wriggle and Siral got up and hit him across the face several times. Hashmat cried, his head shot back and he banged it against the window. He again wriggled and again Siral slapped him across the face. Hashmat cried, looked at me, and quite shocked, I suggested I had Hashmat for a time. Siral assented without expression. Hashmat cried and held on to my neck.

In spite of brutal attacks such as the one I witnessed here, and the limitations of the emotional responsiveness Hashmat received, his development continued in a somewhat covert manner. That this development had continued beneath a disguise of unadventurousness was made vividly apparent by the spurt in his development which coincided with mother's return from hospital. He was walking *and* speaking before his first birthday:

> Javed Ahmed stood Hashmat on the floor and he walked a few steps towards us, and said 'Mama'. Rani, with Fashmat on her lap, looked at him and smiled to me and repeated 'Mama'.

Now he was a mixture of confidence and fragility:

> He walked a couple of steps across the floor – looking fragile, but seeming confident. He looked round and walked across to the sofa, again taking fragile but confident steps.

He emphasised he was no longer the baby by repudiating his drinking bottle:

> Hashmat took the bottle in his hand and tipped it up, letting it drip behind the sofa. Belal stood it up, and Hashmat, standing on Belal's lap, tipped it up again. As it dripped down behind the sofa he called out loudly, 'ahh, ahh, ahh'.

DEVELOPMENT FROM TWELVE TO TWENTY-FOUR MONTHS

In the aftermath of the arrival of Fashmat and the adaptation of the family to another baby, Hashmat was faced with a choice. On the one hand, he could accept the family norm that babies were like fruit, and as common, and that the vulnerable, dependent attitudes of infancy should be abruptly shed. On the other hand, he could struggle to maintain a relationship to his mother, with all that implied in terms of experiencing individuality, uniqueness and the capacity to communicate internal states of mind. The precariousness of this struggle was seen as Hashmat negotiated the passage between these two alternative ways of relating. Suddenly he was a toddler, not a baby. Developmental progress, taking his first steps and saying 'Mama', gave him added capacity and separateness. It also confirmed his 'toddlerhood'. He could now join the 'gang' of brothers.

During this second year he charted a course through three predominant qualities of relationships with others and himself. First, there was a boy who had the capacity to communicate his needs and pain and demonstrate curiosity. He could demand a place with mother and hold on to her (there were occasions when I saw him standing by her, holding his hand on her knee – the hand continued to be important for him). My presence was increasingly linked with this process. He became attached to some of the trappings of my role: my glasses, watch and briefcase. The glasses seemed to symbolise my function. He wore them (in imitation or identification with me) and explored their properties, touching them and looking through them. For example when he was eighteen months eleven days:

> He climbed on the chair and sat next to me. He looked at my face, and then my glasses and he gently leaned over and took them off. He passed them back to me. He took them off and passed them back, and I

put them on. He did this again and put his face to the lens and sucked lightly.

My watch was clearly a symbol of my coming and going. He would come to me at the beginning of observations and ask to wear it. It appeared to help him work through the issue of separation and reunion. He was proprietorial with my briefcase, sitting on it, carrying it around and preventing Fashmat from reaching it. He was most preoccupied with opening it, which he could not. I talked to him a great deal in this second year, and, alongside his increasing curiosity, his language began to develop. He seemed for a time to be bilingual, and his saying 'Oma, Mama' (mother in Bengali and English) appeared apposite. This also amused his mother, Rani, who became capable at times of responding to Hashmat with some concern and protection. These interactions occurred most frequently when Hashmat was in this state of mind – shall I call it that of a family child? – and the parents, watching his play benignly, and with interest, were also in a more 'family' than group mode of relating, usually when the older children were out.

In contrast to this picture, Hashmat's second pattern of relationships was aggressive and sadistic. He joined the 'group' and his attacks focused on Fashmat and the feeding bottle in equal measure. His shifts from one state of mind to the other could happen quite quickly, in the course of a single observation.

Hashmat's third quality of relationships was characterised by a particular kind of withdrawal. He spent periods of time looking out of the window, in a rigid and 'switched off' mode. He became transfixed on these occasions, unaware of my presence, even on the occasions that I held him. This appeared to be a continuation of the development of a withdrawn part of himself, which had been observed from very early in his life, whereby he became mindless in the face of external threats, depending on keeping a low profile in order to survive.

What was particularly interesting from the point of view of the observer's role was how, in the more active role that had developed in this observation I fulfilled the function of helping Hashmat connect his different levels of experience which were observed in these three predominant kinds of relationships with himself and others.

The following sequences from an observation when Hashmat was fifteen months and one week demonstrate both the shift from one part of his self to another, and the observer's role in providing a link between these states of mind. The observation ended with a demonstration of the kind of risk to which Hashmat was vulnerable:

Mother showed Hashmat a tank on the living room floor and moved it, playfully. Hashmat pushed the tank and then stood up. Rani went out and Hashmat looked at me and held his finger in his mouth with a pained expression. I imitated him and asked if it hurt. He smiled and moved his finger round his mouth. He moved across the room and picked up a toy, went to the doorway and picked up a belt and then turned round, looked at me, showed me the belt and went out of the room.

So far he was demonstrating his curiosity through playing and relating.

I followed him and found Shakil and a friend in a bedroom, and Hashmat stood on a chair. They seemed to stop playing as I went in and then carried on. Rani came in behind me and Hashmat picked up a pair of scissors, a large dressmaking pair. Rani reacted with a worried expression, saying 'No, no', and took them from him. He threw some pegs on the floor and then Rani picked him up and carried him into the kitchen. She gave him a tin (baby food) which had a string, making a handle, and some pegs in it. Hashmat took this and threw the pegs on the floor. He came up to me, shaped as if to throw the tin and then passed it to me. I took it and passed it back.

Here there was some modulation; Hashmat appeared to think as he was approaching an attack, and used me to assist in the process of thinking. The observation continued:

He went down the corridor. Shakil and his friend went out to play and Hashmat cried and pointed to the door. He then turned to Rani and reached out to hold her saree. She did not respond and he cried and held his arms higher seeking to be picked up. She did not respond and he turned away and went into the bedroom where there were two bikes. He touched them quite gently and picked up some papers, studied them and then put them down, letting them fall to the floor. He looked up and saw me and moved sideways a few steps until he was out of sight, then he moved back and smiled when I came into view. He looked at me again and walked up to me and touched me on the leg, quite tenderly, and then walked backwards still looking at me until he hit the bed. The force of this knocked him over and he looked quite shocked, on all fours. He stayed there for a moment and then stood up.

During this passage he stayed related to me, with a hint of a 'peek a boo', and tenderness. Provocation followed:

The sound of Fashmat crying came into the room. Hashmat picked up the tin and went out of the room and into the kitchen. Rani called out to him 'No, no, no, hey hey hey'; he followed her into the living room as Fashmat still cried. He climbed up on to the sofa and reached up to his bottle which was resting on the back of the sofa. He turned to me and held the bottle tightly between his teeth, pulling the bottle. Rani looked at him and stood up and fetched a pillow for him, seeming to understand what he wanted. She lay this on the sofa and sat down on the adjacent chair with Fashmat still crying, on her lap. Hashmat lay down on the sofa with the bottle and sucked it. He lifted his left leg up in the air and looked straight ahead and tensed his leg as he held it in the air. He twisted round so he lay on his side still sucking his bottle which he held in his right hand, while his left hand covered his ear. Fashmat stopped crying but Hashmat still covered his ear. He twisted right round so he was lying on his tummy, his head on its side in a contraposta. He was now sucking more air than milk. He turned again and looked at Rani and passed her the bottle.

Hashmat twisted himself in a muscular fashion as he drank. He seemed to struggle with his feelings of being the second baby, sharing mother with Fashmat. Rani retained a connection with him:

Rani held a biro out to him and he climbed to his feet and slid off the sofa, landing on an empty lemonade bottle, crushing it. He exchanged the bottle for the pen and took it to one of the toys on the floor, bent over and started to push the pen into a hole on the surface of the toy. Rani went to answer a knock at the door, carrying Fashmat. Hashmat followed. A friend came in preceded by her little boy, and he went to play with the toys in a bin. Hashmat went up to the boy, and took a toy himself. Then gently and deliberately he hit the other child with it, several times. The boy cried and called his mother's attention. Rani said something to Hashmat and Hashmat got another toy and hit the boy again.

After this attack on the boy, who may be seen to represent the 'baby', Hashmat left the room and I followed him. His state of mind changed and he had become an attacker of other babies, like his brothers. His perspective then appeared to reverse from being the aggressor to being the victim. When he reverted to the victim, he was at risk:

I found him in the bedroom, kneeling on the bed and hanging out of the open window. I put him down on the floor and he protested, then he ran round the bed and came up to me with a smile and then sat next to me and I held him as he looked out of the window. He called out repeatedly 'Mama' pushing the window to and fro. We stayed like this for a time and then as it was time to go I picked him up and he complained as I carried him away from the window. I went to the living room and told Rani he had been hanging out of the window. Rani registered shock and concern and said he was very naughty.

Holding him had helped him verbalise the problem he demonstrated in a concrete way, of feeling, or being, lost and outside. Here was risk with some emphasis, as he became, in his mind, the subject of the attacks on dependency. It seemed quite incongruous that the small, delicate, almost fragile Hashmat could attempt to be so tough. Identification with the older brothers was pronounced by the time he was 2, a consequence it would seem of the constant attacks from the brothers and the event of Fashmat's arrival. He imitated Shakil's tone of voice, the way the older boys brushed their hair, and he got into Miral's shoes, literally:

> Hashmat had left the room and now he came back in wearing big brother Miral's shoes. He grinned broadly and then seriously tried to concentrate on walking in them. (Hashmat at twenty-two months six days)

Hashmat is not only trying the shoes on for fun, he is aspiring to the position they represent, namely, a position of strength in the family, and toughness. Toughness is commonly the defence of the deprived child (see, for example, Williams 1984). In this observation, Belal, the 10-year-old, told the family story in the form of an allegory of the consequences of there being so many children:

> Belal sat on the chair by the table and told me a story about finding a golden eagle in the flat opposite; the eagle had many babies and they fought each other. The eagle had bitten his hand and he had to go to hospital. He was having to go to stay with his cousin for two weeks because he had been in trouble for tearing the wallpaper off the wall. He was in trouble for fighting here but he would fight with his cousins there and be in trouble again.

In the conflict between the siblings, humour and deadliness could follow upon one another. When the movement was from deadliness to humour, a sense of horseplay was introduced instead of grievous bodily harm. This was exemplified by Hashmat's fight with Shakil when he was eighteen months and twenty-five days:

> Hashmat followed Shakil, calling 'Oma' and 'uhh'. Gritting his teeth he hit Shakil on the back and arm. Shakil pretended to be dead and lay on the chair. Hashmat watched him and then hit him several times on the back, as if to stir him. Shakil got up with a big grin.

I found that as the observations continued, and as the two boys played out their fights, I became less antagonised by the behaviour. I could say that my counter-transference changed, moved by Shakil's humour. It was possible to differentiate between a playful, humorous event and its vicious counterpart, a violent enactment. I wondered in particular how toughness, the capacity to fight, to maintain a possession, or even one's own body boundaries, was crucial to the existence of young Asian boys living in contemporary British society.

The end of the observation, after two years, was difficult to contemplate, and to work with. It was painful to think of ending and Hashmat had a significant attachment to me. On one occasion, at twenty-two months two weeks, in an act reminiscent of 'John' in the Robertsons' film (Robertson and Robertson 1969) he put on his coat and shoes as I was leaving. With much repetition, there was some working through before the end of the observations. The last observation, two days after his second birthday was a moving occasion, where Hashmat joined me in a meal:

> Rani cleared the table and invited me to sit there. Hashmat looked up at me and called me 'Moma'. Rani laughed and spoke to Miral who told me Hashmat was calling me 'uncle'. Rani said: 'Bengali "oma"; English "mama"; English "uncle", Bengali "moma" '. Hashmat looked up at me eating and then pulled a chair for himself and sat on it. Rani gave him a plate and he ate his rice and curry with his fingers. He pointed to the water jug and I poured him some water in the glass. He drank some and pointed again and I refilled it for him. He raised his glass and I raised mine and he said 'Cheers'. I said 'Cheers' and we touched glasses. This was repeated several times, each time he said 'Cheers' and smiled at me.

CONCLUSION

In this chapter I have concentrated on an observation of an infant, Hashmat, who was one of the five infants at potential risk in the sample I studied. In following his development over the two-year period I was able to observe how he moved between times and situations of risk and times where he gathered greater resilience. The problems he faced have been described in terms of the quality of the patterns of containment provided by all the family members. At times it was necessary for his survival to adopt a very withdrawn form of adaptation. In spurts, and almost covertly, his development continued, so that by the end of the two-year period there were some encouraging features to observe and describe. In the course of observing in a setting which was cross-cultural and initially provided difficulties in communication, I adapted the traditional observational role, to one in which there was a form of purposeful activity, not initiating interaction, but responding in a way I have summarised as 'auxiliary parenting'. This led to a complex relationship developing between Hashmat and myself which made a contribution to the quality of his development.

REFERENCES

Bick, E. (1968) 'The Experience of the skin in early object relations', *International Journal of Psycho-Analysis*, 49: 484–486.

Bion, W. R. (1962) *Learning from Experience*, London: Heinemann.

Briggs, S. (1996) 'An intensive observational study of five infants at potential risk', Ph.D. Thesis, University of East London.

Briggs, S. (1997) *Growth and Risk in Infancy*, London: Jessica Kingsley.

Robertson, J. and Robertson, J. (1969) *Young Children in Brief Separation*, Ipswich: Concord Films.

Murray, L. and Trevarthen, C. (1986) 'The infant's role in mother–infant communication', *Journal of Child Language*, 13: 15–29.

Watson, J. (ed.) (1977) *Between Two Cultures*, Oxford: Blackwell.

Henry Williams, G. (1984) 'Difficulties about thinking and learning', in M. Boston and R. Szur (eds) *Psychotherapy with Severely Deprived Children*, London: Routledge and Kegan Paul.

Endpiece

Susan Reid

It seems impossible, once exposed, to resist the pull of infant observation. Many students find the impact on their professional work, on the understanding of human emotional growth and development, and the obstacles to it, the most important learning experience they have. At the Tavistock Clinic students from a wide range of professional backgrounds are engaged in observing infants; they come from child psychotherapy; adult psychotherapy; child, adolescent and adult psychiatry; social work, clinical and educational psychology; the probation service; psychiatric nursing; speech therapy; music therapy; teaching; art therapy; nursery workers and other professions.

As outlined in this book, students from abroad who trained at the Tavistock have taken this exciting new experience home to their countries of origin, where it has been adapted to suit a range of training needs for different professional groups. It has been used to influence positive changes in clinical practice, for example, in premature baby units and paediatric clinics. The same methodology has been adapted for observations of other age groups and in a variety of settings. In Great Britain, infant observation has gradually, steadily, infiltrated many professional trainings until it becomes difficult to find a mental health training which does not include it. The requests for someone to teach infant observation to a new group seem inexhaustible. Nowadays it can be difficult, in London, to find a baby to observe; there are so many students seeking out families who will allow them this privilege!

Such a source of information about human development was unlikely to remain a secret for long, indeed it is clear that no one who becomes involved in infant observation wishes it to be so. It becomes a passion, and a passion practitioners wish to share. It is the wish to share this passion which has brought this book into being. We hope the reader who has not observed an infant before, may be stimulated to do so. For all readers we hope the book will have stimulated an interest in the many applications of this methodology.

Index